Safe Medicine for Sober People

ALSO BY GENE HAWES

*Addiction Free: How to Help an Alcoholic or Addict
Get Started on Recovery* (WITH ANDERSON HAWES)

*Rx for Recovery: The Medical and Health Guide for Alcoholics,
Addicts, and Their Families* (WITH JEFFREY WEISBERG, M.D.)

Childbearing: A Book of Choices (WITH DR. RUTH WATSON LUBIC)

The Career-Changer's Sourcebook

The College Board Guide to Going to College While Working

The Encyclopedia of Second Careers

Hawes on Getting into College

Hawes Guide to Successful Study Skills (WITH LYNNE S. HAWES)

Hawes Comprehensive Guide to Colleges

The Complete Career Guide (WITH DAVID M. BROWNSTONE)

Careers Tomorrow: Leading Growth Fields for College Graduates

The New American Guide to Colleges

How to Get College Scholarships

*To Advance Knowledge: A Handbook on American
University Press Publishing*

Educational Testing for the Millions

THOMAS DUNNE BOOKS
ST. MARTIN'S GRIFFIN
NEW YORK

Safe Medicine

for

Sober People

HOW TO AVOID RELAPSING
ON PAIN, SLEEP, COLD, OR
ANY OTHER MEDICATION

Jeffrey Weisberg, M.D.

and

Gene Hawes

Disclaimer

The information about the drugs contained herein is general in nature and is intended to be used in consultation with your health-care providers. It is not intended to replace specific instructions, directions, or warnings given to you by your physician or other prescriber, or accompanying a particular product. The information is selective and it is not claimed that it includes all known precautions, contraindications, effects, or interactions possibly related to the use of a drug. The information may differ from that contained in the product labeling that is required by law. The information is not sufficient to make an evaluation as to the risks and benefits of taking a particular drug in a particular case, is not medical advice for individual problems, and should not alone be relied upon for these purposes. Since the inclusion or exclusion of particular information about a drug is judgmental in nature and since opinion as to drug usage may differ, you may wish to consult additional sources. Should you desire additional information, or if you have any questions as to how this information may relate to you in particular, ask your doctor, nurse, pharmacist, or other health-care provider. The publisher is not advocating the use of any product described in this book, does not warrant or guarantee any of these products, and has not performed any independent analysis in connection with the product information contained herein.

THOMAS DUNNE BOOKS.
An imprint of St. Martin's Press.

www.stmartins.com

ISBN 0-312-30547-8

First Edition: April 2005

D   10   9   8   7   6   5   4   3   2

Contents

Acknowledgments

Clinical experience, research in relevant literature, and a great many interviews with individuals recovering from alcoholism, drug addiction, or both were among the sources we used in writing *Safe Medicine for Sober People*. Many interviews were carried out with members of Alcoholics Anonymous and such related recovery programs as Narcotics Anonymous and Cocaine Anonymous.

The book also relies heavily on case histories of individuals treated by Dr. Weisberg. However, details of those identified herein as alcoholics/addicts have been altered to render them unrecognizable. We have done this both to protect the confidentiality of the physician-patient relationship, and to support the principle of anonymity in AA and other recovery programs. To each person whose experience contributes so invaluably to the book, we are immensely grateful.

Certain individuals who can be identified helped us in special ways. Barbara Stanton, a credentialed alcoholism counselor, was wonderfully generous in providing much essential advice and interview material. Harrison Evarts aided with the research and drafting of portions of Chapter 3, "Safe—and Highly Unsafe—Medicines in Recovery." Extensive compilation, drafting, and editing of material in that chapter were carried out with high competence by Catherine Settens. To each of these individuals, our heartfelt thanks.

Organizations and agencies were also most generous and cooperative in providing information. These include Alcoholics Anonymous World Services Office, the central office of the National Council on Alcoholism and Drug Dependence, Al-Anon Family Groups Headquarters, the American Society of Addiction Medicine, the American Academy of Addiction Psychiatry, the Center of Alcohol Studies at Rutgers University, the National Institute on Alcohol Abuse and Alcoholism, the National Institute on Drug Abuse, and the Substance Abuse and Mental Health Services Administration.

In the creation of this book, Thomas Dunne and Marcia Markland, both of St. Martin's Press, have played literally indispensable roles.

To all these and others who helped, we express our grateful appreciation.

Preface

The behavioral and physical deterioration in alcoholism and drug addiction are so alike that we often use the term *addiction* in referring to both. We know that recovery from addiction—the compulsive and physical need to repetitively ingest a substance— requires abstinence. The sometimes subtle steps leading to the relapse of the recovering addict must be fiercely guarded against. Among those precarious steps, the inadvertent ingestion of certain medications has often been seen to trigger relapse.

Clinical experience has taught me that the alcoholic or addict is never cured. His or her addiction can only be arrested and placed in a state of remission. Abstinence is the first step: the recovering addict can never again take a mood-altering substance without risk to his or her sobriety. This sobriety is so critical that the recovering addict must take extreme care with medical issues and medications. As a doctor, I have often fielded questions regarding the medical aspects of recovery. I have paid close attention to the clinical course of active addiction and to the nature of recovery. It is clear that a reference book is needed to help explain where, in the world of medications and medical care, there is danger for the recovering alcoholic or addict.

It was years ago that I first became aware of an underground epidemic. As an emergency-medicine specialist in the 1970s, I treated acute intoxication, drug overdoses, drug-induced psychiatric catastrophes, alcohol withdrawal, convulsions, delirium tremens, drug-related trauma, cocaine psychosis, alcoholic cardiac and liver disease, narcotic-induced respiratory arrest, drug-related family crises, acute esophageal hemorrhage, and on and on. I was constantly faced with desperate people locked in their addictions. Some pretended to have physical ailments in order to obtain prescription drugs; others became victims of tragic disability and death as the result of untethered drug and alcohol abuse.

At that time, there seemed to be little awareness of—or focus on—the source of all this human chaos. The medical world saw hepatitis, broken bones, and withdrawal symptoms. More socially oriented professionals saw placement problems, family disorder, and domestic abuse. Cultural critics discussed the reasons for increased "recreational" drug use—and the suffering continued.

As my career progressed, I had the opportunity to participate in organizing an alcohol and drug rehabilitation program. This gave me my first insight into alcoholism and drug addiction as primary pathology. My clinical interest was awakened, and over the years since then, I have observed and treated alcoholics and drug addicts with ever-increasing interest and understanding.

I have worked with alcoholism and drug counselors, consulted with recovering alcoholics and addicts, and explored the literature. But more than any of this, the clinical arena has been where my ideas, understanding, and positions have taken form. I have formulated my views of alcoholism and drug addiction from observing patients and others over the years, and from listening carefully to their stories.

The public has certainly come to recognize alcoholism and drug addiction as a ubiqitous affliction, and recovery programs are now considered essential for those afflicted.

The ever-expanding recovering community needs more accessible answers regarding matters of vital interest. Gene Hawes and I agreed that such information would be valuable, not only to recovering people themselves, but to their families, their physicians, and everyone with any involvement in alcoholism or drug addiction.

Jeffrey Weisberg, M.D.

One

Safeguarding Recovery:

THE MEDICAL
FUNDAMENTALS

L et's start with an irrefutable observation: alcoholism and drug
addiction destroy lives and wreak havoc on families. Anyone
involved with an addict and anyone hearing the myriad of personal accounts told in treatment programs around the world can
attest to this.

Is addiction a disease? We think so, but whether or not the
term *disease* is accepted, there is no denying that alcoholism and
drug addiction damage a person's organ systems and physiologic
processes while causing emotional and mental deterioration.

Almost magically, though, abstinence and recovery reverse the
physical and emotional deterioration. The addict is returned to
normal life and physical health returns in months, as long as per-
manent damage has not occurred. Emotional and mental health
have a more variable but generally positive course.

All is lost, however, if the addict returns to drinking or using
drugs. In fact, with renewed drinking or drug use, there is an ugly

and rapid return of physical and emotional deterioration, along with immediate physical craving and addiction.

So recovery must be protected fiercely. Recovery programs—most prominently, Alcoholics Anonymous—deal with the complexities of the recovery process. In this book, we treat one area of treachery for the recovering addict: the dangerous area of interaction with the medical world.

Prescription and nonprescription drugs are part of almost everyone's life. However, for people in recovery, some of these medications are dangerous, as they can increase the likelihood of relapse. Thus in this book we examine prescription and nonprescription medications with regard to their mood-altering potential and their risk to the recovering addict. We intend this to serve as a resource for recovering addicts, their family members, and clinicians.

Active alcoholism or drug addiction has a predictable course. Once recognized, the prognosis is clear: deterioration is chronic, progressive, and in the end, usually fatal. Indeed, other diseases are often less predictable.

For example, I recall a patient, Phil W., who came to me with a swollen knee. Blood tests indicated he had rheumatoid arthritis. When Phil asked what he could expect as time went on, I told him that symmetrical joints usually develop pain and swelling of varying degrees. There are medicines and physical measures to help, I said, but often deformity results. I did say that every situation is different, however, and we'd just have to wait and see. Luckily, the swelling in Phil's knee went down within two weeks, and he has had no symptoms of rheumatoid arthritis since. That was eight years ago.

However, had Phil come to me with a deteriorating marriage and depression related to drinking too much, I could have predicted his future much more accurately. "If you continue to drink," I would have said, "your marriage will become unsalvageable. You'll become isolated and lonely, filled with self-disgust and fear. You will begin to drink every night until you pass out, and there will be nothing in your life besides work and drinking. You won't have any fun in life; you'll be besieged by problems that seem insurmountable, and soon you'll have trouble at work. Your liver tests will show alcoholic hepatitis; you'll develop gastritis or ulcers, and then more serious consequences. Finally, if you keep drinking, in time there will be a critical or fatal event, either a medical catastrophe or a fatal accident."

This clinical predictability is uncannily accurate. We invariably see a complex pattern of emotional and physical circumstances that leads to a compulsion to drink a toxic chemical. This then sets up a cascade of events that, without fail, results in the deterioration of one's physical, social, and emotional health.

The hereditary character of alcoholism is clear. A classic forty-five-year study of alcoholism found that more than three times as many men with relatives who abuse alcohol developed alcohol dependence, compared to men with no relatives who abuse alcohol. (This was reported in *The Natural History of Alcoholism* by George E. Vaillant in 1983.) Another study analyzed alcoholism among two groups of Danish men who had been adopted in early infancy by nonrelatives. One group consisted of men with at least one alcoholic biological parent. The second group consisted of men with biological parents who were not alcoholics. Four times as many men with an alcoholic parent became alcoholics. In addition, there was no consistent relationship between alcoholism in adoptive parents and alcoholism in the adopted sons, thus suggesting that environmental factors were inconsequential compared to hereditary factors. (Donald W. Goodwin, F. Schulsinger, L. Hermansen, S. B. Guze, and G. Winokur, "Alcohol Problems in Adoptees Raised Apart From Biological Parents," *Archives of General Psychiatry,*

1973, 28:238–243.) In all, more than one hundred scientific studies confirming the genetic character of alcoholism have been made.

Most diseases are usually first recognized in their most severe or pronounced form. Later, more subtle and less severe forms of the disease are recognized, and soon the disease has a much broader definition. Eventually, scientific research establishes diagnostic parameters for a given disease (laboratory tests, X-ray findings, and the like), and then, when possible, a cause, or *etiology,* is uncovered. A treatment or cure may be found at the same time.

The process whereby we first discover and then learn successively more and more about a disease is happening with alcoholism. At first, only the most hopeless, extreme cases were recognized as alcoholics. In the 1930s, when Alcoholics Anonymous (AA) was established, these extreme cases served as the model of the disease.

Since then, less extreme cases with varying patterns of drinking have broadened the concept of the disease of alcoholism. The American Medical Association first officially defined alcoholism as a disease in 1956. A recent revision of the official diagnostic manual of the American Psychiatric Association specified three main criteria for the diagnosis of alcohol or drug dependency:

1. the suffering of withdrawal symptoms after intake is stopped,
2. the need for ingesting constantly increased quantities in order to realize the desired effect,
3. an obsession with alcohol or drugs so severe that it leads to taking risks to obtain them and seriously interferes with work and social life.

Other organizations that define alcoholism as a disease include the American College of Physicians, the American Hospital Association, the American Public Health Association, the American

Psychological Association, the National Association of Social Workers, and the World Health Organization.

There are several ways to view alcoholism, but as a clinical entity, it can be described as a maladaptive and self-destructive behavior pattern involving the compulsive consumption of alcohol leading to personal, emotional, and physical deterioration. This behavior is associated with excessive fear, depression, and anxiety, and a resulting difficulty in coping with the normal stresses of life.

Alcoholism is also characterized by varying degrees of toxic damage brought on by excessive consumption. Alcohol is, of course, toxic to the nonalcoholic as well as to the alcoholic. As a drug, it is absorbed directly through the stomach wall or the walls of the small intestine and passes quickly into the bloodstream. It then moves into every part of the body that contains water. Five percent of it is eliminated through the breath, urine, or sweat, but the remaining 95 percent must be broken down by the liver. The liver processes alcohol at the rate of about one-third ounce of ethanol (pure 200-proof alcohol) per hour. Any more than this continues to circulate in the blood and the cells.

Within a few minutes, alcohol reaches the brain, where it initially stimulates and agitates but eventually acts as a depressant. First, the functions of inhibition and judgment are depressed, which accounts for the release of normal restraint. Sexual inhibitions, for example, may initially be relaxed, but alcohol actually impairs sexual function, performance, and eventually desire. Mood changes are severe with intoxication, and some people suffer Jekyll-and-Hyde personality changes.

Alcohol then affects motor ability, reaction time, eyesight, and other functions, and if there is continued intake, vital functions can be affected and death can occur. Usually the body rejects the alcohol by vomiting first; later it may become comatose before a fatal dose can be consumed.

Because alcohol reaches every cell and organ of the body, its physical effects are wide-ranging. When chronic alcohol intake persists, the result is metabolic damage everywhere: in the liver, the central nervous system, the gastrointestinal system, and the heart. Other effects include impaired vision, impaired sexual function, circulation problems, malnutrition, water retention, pancreatitis, skin disorders (such as acne and dilation of blood vessels), muscle atrophy, and decreased resistance to infection.

The liver is the most common site of alcohol toxicity. First, *fatty liver,* an infiltration of the liver with abnormal fatty cells, occurs, producing general liver enlargement. Next comes *alcoholic hepatitis,* in which the cells are injured and some die. Further alcohol exposure eventually causes *cirrhosis,* the irreversible destruction of liver cells and fibrous scarring of the entire liver. Obstruction of the flow of blood through the liver and deterioration of liver function result. Many bodily functions are disturbed by each of these liver diseases, and death results in 10 to 30 percent of cases.

Alcohol reduces the amount of oxygen reaching the brain and destroys brain cells directly. With chronic abuse, an individual may experience seizures, as well as neurologic disorders characterized by dementia, such as *Korsakoff's syndrome.* Its symptoms include amnesia, disorientation, hallucinations, emotional disturbances, and loss of muscle control.

The digestive system suffers various injuries when alcohol abuse is chronic. Inflammation of the esophagus and stomach (that is, esophagitis and gastritis) occurs, and there is an increased incidence of ulcers. Indirectly, the blood vessels in the esophagus dilate due to obstruction of blood flow in the portal system of the liver. This can lead to a fatal hemorrhage.

With alcoholism, there is also an increased frequency of cancer, both in the liver and upper gastrointestinal organs (such as the esophagus). In addition, the heart is affected directly by a disease of the heart muscle called *cardiomyopathy,* and indirectly by high blood pressure and arrhythmias.

Alcoholism is relentlessly progressive. That is, as long as drinking continues, all symptoms steadily worsen. The rate of the destructive progression varies, often with long periods of slow decline and then sudden periods of much more rapid deterioration. Every case is somewhat different from the next.

Some alcoholics begin drinking abnormally from their first drink, behaving from the beginning in ways destructive to their health. For others, there is a period of acceptable social drinking. Perhaps there are a few "drunks" and related hangovers, but on looking back, it would be difficult to distinguish the early alcoholic from the social drinker. Indeed, most alcoholics have had an early period when there was still some fun in their drinking.

Sooner or later, however, the alcoholic begins to inappropriately use alcohol or drugs for their mood-altering qualities. In the early stages, perhaps the drinking is limited to recreational, or "reward," periods. That is, the individual is still working well and handling life adequately, but weekends are characterized by needing some form of escaping or decreasing tension. Drinking or drugging becomes the chief activity of nonworking recreational time. Activities are chosen subconsciously because they involve drinking or drugging. Gradually the alcoholic will socialize mainly or only with others who drink; he'll plan dinners and events that involve drinking, such as visits to restaurants suited to several cocktails and wine with dinner, family outings to pizza parlors where having a pitcher of beer is appropriate, or trips to sports events where beer is plentiful.

In time, all recreational activity probably has some relationship to drinking, and the alcoholic comes to depend more and more on the mood-altering qualities of the drug. A drink is needed to relax, to celebrate, to mourn, to welcome the weekend. Soon the special occasion is any occasion.

At this stage, the alcoholic begins to feel anxious and uncomfortable with many of life's normal activities. He may need a few quick drinks to get ready for a party or social engagement. He may even avoid social activities in favor of staying home and drinking in front of the TV or going to his favorite bar.

Some alcoholics may consciously control the number of drinks they allow themselves (for instance, "no more than two before dinner"). As time goes on, however, alcoholics find their drinking time to be increasingly important. They may make it through the workday without drinking, but they begin to get tense toward afternoon and sometimes even become obsessed with the idea of getting home, where they are able to drink. The compulsion to get the first drink of the day increases. The first drink may move into the workday and to an earlier hour on the weekends.

Although the tolerance for alcohol may become high, the alcoholic begins to have more periods of drunkenness and soon has blackouts (periods of memory loss). For example, during a blackout, Terry C. drove from San Francisco, California, to Reno, Nevada, and got married, not remembering any of it afterward. Some alcoholics are not aware of blackouts, however, because they don't have anyone around to describe the forgotten events.

By this time, there are usually significant problems as a result of alcoholism. The alcoholic may feel depressed and may think he drinks because of depression. During this phase, many alcoholics try psychotherapy, but because they deny their drinking problem, they usually get little help. They know something is wrong, but their drinking seems secondary, a response to anxiety and depression. They can't see drinking as the primary problem.

Marital problems, social problems, and health problems may now be part of the picture. The alcoholic at this stage is having no fun. He is desperately trying to avoid the pain he doesn't understand. Only drinking does the trick, briefly. But the pain returns daily. Anxiety, tearfulness, difficulty making it through each day, and a sense of doom and failure characterize his life.

The drink or drug now sets up a craving for more, and matters are totally out of control. Awful things sometimes happen at this point: a spouse may leave, a serious accident may occur, a job may be lost. Something can easily happen to bring on "the bottom." The alcoholic's bottom is that point of such hopelessness and desperation that he will do anything to change and will even consider that the drinking itself may be the problem. There is now a crack, however small, in the alcoholic's denial.

This progression is a general description. Many alcoholics go through long periods of trying to control their drinking or even attempting to stop. Without recovery programs, however, this rarely helps. The emotional part of the disease persists during self-imposed attempts at control or abstinence, and eventually the progression picks up steam again. Active alcoholics attempt to control their progression in varying ways. Many switch from liquor to beer or to wine or even to other drugs, convincing themselves that this may solve their problem. Sometimes they give up drinking to prove they are not alcoholics, but take Valium or other drugs instead, and the disease presses on. Others try a "geographic cure," moving to a new state or a new job to start over. These are desperate attempts to treat the confusing, painful turmoil in their lives. They still can't see alcohol or drugs as the primary problem. Denial is an extremely strong mechanism in addiction.

Denial tells the alcoholic that alcohol is not his problem. Although he is caught in a tumultous array of troubles all linked to his drinking, denial allows the alcoholic to blame everything but drinking for them. Drinking is rationalized to be the result of his problems, not the cause. The alcoholic thinks he gets drunk because of stress, depression, situations at work, unfairness, and the like.

Toward the end, everyone suffers. The alcoholic blames everyone around him and spreads his self-centered misery to each family member, even though he may not wish to.

At the end, there is an alcoholic who loathes himself, who is constantly miserable and crawling out of his skin with trembling anxiety, and who is isolated from the world and profoundly depressed. Suicide may enter his mind. He is obsessed with alcohol and will keep drinking, possibly around the clock, despite the pleading of those close to him. Health problems, lost job, lost family, and even legal problems may be part of the picture. Often alcoholics reach the state of being too sick to drink and too sick not to drink. Withdrawal symptoms, ranging from shakes to delirium to convulsions, surface when alcohol cannot be absorbed. The alcoholic is a physical wreck, and if he does not begin recovery at this point, he will end up hospitalized or dead. Today, though, recovery programs have become widespread, and most recovering alcoholics/addicts begin their sobriety before experiencing these end-stage symptoms.

For some reason, it seems that "the bottom" must be reached for alcoholic recovery to begin. It is important to realize, however, that the bottom need not be the absolute end of the road. In fact, many alcoholics hit bottom long before they have serious disruptions in their health or careers. To some, the bottom may come when they are confronted by their boss; to others, it may be the acting-out of their children. *High bottom* and *low bottom* are terms that refer to two differing levels of alcoholic progression needed for denial to be pierced and recovery to begin.

Unfortunately, many alcoholics never find recovery. They die, or become permanently brain-injured psychiatric-hospital inmates, or go on living at the bottom. These are all horrifying tragedies.

We have referred to the compulsive drive to drink as one of the benchmarks in alcoholism. The alcoholic reaches a stage where one drink creates a craving for another, and consequently the typical alcoholic pattern eventually includes daily drinking. There is another pattern, however, which deserves mention: that of the periodic alcoholic, who does not drink daily but who has drinking bouts of varying frequency. He may drink once a month or just a few times a year. Each episode, however, usually produces drunkenness and demonstrates the person's powerlessness over the drink. The periodic alcoholic is often just as sick as the daily drinker. However, his denial may be even stronger since there are long stretches of abstinence to convince the drinker that he doesn't have a problem.

Progression is another characteristic of alcoholism. When an alcoholic begins drinking, his tolerance for alcohol and the strength of his compulsion are both low. As his drinking goes on through the years, both the tolerance and the compulsion increase. In late stages, the tolerance falls, but the compulsion remains strong. Therefore, a very late-stage alcoholic may have an irrepressible compulsion to drink but may have blackouts and become quite sick after just a few drinks. Years earlier he could probably have held a fifth of vodka without any problem. Observing those who have relapsed, a fascinating picture of this progression appears. It may continue even if the alcoholic stops drinking. Alcoholics who had been sober for years, but who eventually started drinking again, found that their tolerance was the same or lower, and their compulsion the same or stronger than it had been previously.

Carl C. started drinking in college, where he was one of those who could down tremendous quantities of beer. He later became a journalist, and his alcoholism progressed through the years. At first his drinking was limited to evenings at home, but eventually he was having several drinks at lunch. In time, he was hiding bottles in his office and at home and drinking up to one and a half fifths of vodka per day. As his disease progressed, he lost his family and was hospitalized several times with painful pancreatitis. Finally, after twenty years of abuse, Carl would get sick and black out after drinking only half a pint. Sometimes he couldn't even drink that much without getting sick. He was in a constant state of illness and withdrawal when an old friend convinced him to go to a detoxification and rehabilitation program.

Carl became sober and stayed with an AA recovery program. Things went well after a while. He established a rather normal life. Eight years later he became extremely angry over something that happened at work. He became obsessed by it, and one night he went to a local restaurant and had a drink before dinner. Feeling that the drink had caused him no problem, he had two more—and he didn't remember anything that occurred after that. Apparently, Carl went into a blackout, was taken home by a friend, and passed out for the night. The next day he had an awful hangover, but by afternoon he drank again, only to have the same scenario repeat itself. After two weeks of this torture, Carl suffered a convulsion and was taken to a hospital detoxification program, where he stayed five days before being transferred to a rehabilitation program. Realizing the inevitable horror of returning to alcohol, Carl then committed himself to AA with new intensity.

Carl's story is not unique. Many stories illustrate the mysterious fact that the progression of the disease, as measured by physical tolerance, can march on even during periods of abstinence. Carl's experience also points out that the compulsion is triggered by the first exposure to alcohol, even after years of abstention.

Carl's experience, and that of thousands like him, also points out the most basic and important principle of recovery: this disease can be arrested only with complete abstinence. There are no cures, and as AA wisely observes, it's the first drink that makes the alcoholic drunk, not the tenth.

When alcoholics/addicts become so desperate that their denial begins to weaken, there is a chance they will accept some form of help. Sometimes it is a severe health problem that prompts this acceptance; sometimes it is a formal intervention; sometimes it is the urging of a relative or friend; and sometimes the addict seeks help on his own. At this point, recovery may begin, but the road ahead is not necessarily smooth.

Once he accepts the need to stop drinking, the alcoholic begins the journey into recovery by first undergoing detoxification. At this point most alcoholics are not aware that their disease involves much more than drinking. If they continue into recovery, they will be surprised to learn that it includes an attitude and mood disorder creating psychologic and social dysfunction. The alcoholic or addict will slowly become aware of how comprehensive his recovery must be.

First, however, is detoxification, or acute withdrawal, as the body is forced to acclimate to a new environment and find a physiologic balance in the absence of the drug that has bathed every tissue for so long. Although bodily changes continue for a long time after the alcoholic stops drinking, the acute detox period lasts from three to seven days after complete alcohol abstinence begins.

Symptoms of withdrawal are usually significant and can be life-threatening. They include disorientation, acute anxiety and fear, auditory and visual hallucinations, insomnia, shakiness, agitation, profuse perspiration, rapid pulse, abdominal cramps, diarrhea, and sometimes vomiting. A feeling of internal tremors is often described. More dangerous symptoms include fever, delirium tremens, and convulsions or epileptic seizures.

After the detoxification period, physical and emotional discomforts may continue through many weeks or even many months. Physical difficulties may include insomnia, headaches, and minor but nagging aches and pains in various parts of the body. Among emotional troubles may be extreme mood swings, anxiety, nervous tension, continuing depression, restlessness, and boredom. Health professionals who work with recovering alcoholics and addicts sometimes call such discomforts early in recovery *protracted withdrawal syndrome.*

The other drugs of abuse (such as cocaine, narcotics, tranquilizers, and barbiturates) all have varying acute withdrawal or detoxification intervals, depending somewhat on the amount of chronic intake and the duration of the addiction. Symptoms for all drugs are not identical. Narcotics withdrawal, for instance, involves long periods of marked general discomfort, depression, abdominal and muscle cramps, and periods of extreme agitation, whereas barbiturate withdrawal can include dangerous seizure activity. Valium withdrawal entails long-lasting and profound mood swings.

This stressful period of detoxification is preferably spent under medical supervision. The hospital (specifically its detox ward) is the most common site for such supervision. Some hospital detox programs are integrated with treatment programs or rehabilitation centers, and some operate independently.

More recently, some drug and alcohol counselors, in cooperation with experienced physicians, have been able to design "ambulatory" detoxification programs for appropriate individuals. This, of course, must be done carefully and on a selective basis, but it is an option available in many parts of the country. In such cases, the alcoholic/addict is seen by the counselor and the doctor as an outpatient. He is usually observed daily for the acute period of withdrawal, and less frequently thereafter until he is safely involved in a recovery program such as AA or NA (Narcotics Anonymous).

The detoxification period is indeed the first step in recovery from alcoholism. During this time mental functions are cloudy and concentration is difficult. It is after detox that the alcoholic or addict must begin to focus on the principles of recovery. His success will depend on his commitment to those principles from that time on.

The alcoholic/addict will learn that he will always be in the process of recovery. He will discover that his disease can only be arrested and held in remission. It cannot, at least with present knowledge, be cured. Nevertheless, with the disease in remission, the alcoholic or addict can live a full life, normal in every respect except that he can never take a drink or mood-altering substance again, except under specially supervised medical circumstances. (These exceptions are discussed in later chapters.)

Two diagrams on the accompanying pages summarize in visual form the downward swing marking the progression of alcoholism/addiction, the bottom, and the upward swing of those victims fortunate enough to recover. Figure 1 depicts the progression for the alcoholic or addict, and Figure 2 depicts the progression for family members or others close to the alcoholic or addict. Reprint permission granted by Seabrook House, Seabrook, New Jersey. Copyright 1986 by Seabrook House.

Figure 1, widely used in alcoholism/addiction treatment programs, is called the *Jellinek chart* or the *Max Glatt chart*. Its downward swing to a bottom was developed by E. M. Jellinek, whose definition of alcoholism as a disease in the 1940s was later adopted by the World Health Organization. The chart's upward swing in recovery was developed by M. M. Glatt and introduced in "Group Therapy in Alcoholism," *British Journal of Addiction,* Vol. 54, No. 2, 1957–1959 (according to the Library of the Center for Alcohol Studies at Rutgers, the State University of New Jersey).

Cross-Addiction or Dual Addiction

In this book, we often refer to alcoholics and drug addicts interchangeably. Indeed, many alcoholics in our present culture also use other drugs, and many drug addicts abuse alcohol as well. In fact, as indicated by our survey of rehabilitation centers (see Appendix), a majority of those entering treatment today are addicted

Chemical Dependency & Its Progression

TO BE READ FROM LEFT TO RIGHT

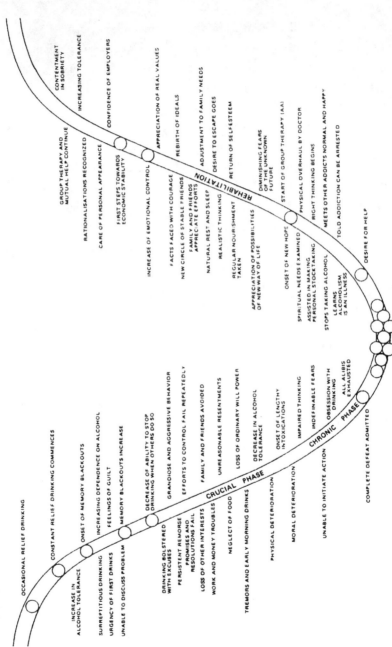

OCCASIONAL RELIEF DRINKING

CONSTANT RELIEF DRINKING COMMENCES

INCREASE IN ALCOHOL TOLERANCE

ONSET OF MEMORY BLACKOUTS

SURREPTITIOUS DRINKING

INCREASING DEPENDENCE ON ALCOHOL

URGENCY OF FIRST DRINKS

FEELINGS OF GUILT

UNABLE TO DISCUSS PROBLEM

MEMORY BLACKOUTS INCREASE

DECREASE OF ABILITY TO STOP DRINKING WHEN OTHERS DO SO

DRINKING BOLSTERED WITH EXCUSES

GRANDIOSE AND AGGRESSIVE BEHAVIOR

PERSISTENT REMORSE

EFFORTS TO CONTROL FAIL REPEATEDLY

PROMISES AND RESOLUTIONS FAIL

FAMILY AND FRIENDS AVOIDED

LOSS OF OTHER INTERESTS

UNREASONABLE RESENTMENTS

WORK AND MONEY TROUBLES

NEGLECT OF FOOD

LOSS OF ORDINARY WILL POWER

TREMORS AND EARLY MORNING DRINKS

DECREASE IN ALCOHOL TOLERANCE

PHYSICAL DETERIORATION

ONSET OF LENGTHY INTOXICATIONS

MORAL DETERIORATION

IMPAIRED THINKING

INDEFINABLE FEARS

UNABLE TO INITIATE ACTION

OBSESSION WITH DRINKING

ALL ALIBIS EXHAUSTED

COMPLETE DEFEAT ADMITTED

CRUCIAL PHASE

CHRONIC PHASE

OBSESSIVE DRINKING CONTINUES IN VICIOUS CIRCLES

LEARNS ALCOHOLISM IS AN ILLNESS

STOPS TAKING ALCOHOL

ASSISTED IN MAKING PERSONAL STOCKTAKING

SPIRITUAL NEEDS EXAMINED

DESIRE FOR HELP

APPRECIATION OF POSSIBILITIES OF NEW WAY OF LIFE

REGULAR NOURISHMENT TAKEN

REALISTIC THINKING

NATURAL REST AND SLEEP

FAMILY AND FRIENDS APPRECIATE EFFORTS

NEW CIRCLE OF STABLE FRIENDS

FACTS FACED WITH COURAGE

INCREASE OF EMOTIONAL CONTROL

TOLD ADDICTION CAN BE ARRESTED

MEETS OTHER ADDICTS NORMAL AND HAPPY

RIGHT THINKING BEGINS

PHYSICAL OVERHAUL BY DOCTOR

START OF GROUP THERAPY (AA)

ONSET OF NEW HOPE

DIMINISHING FEARS OF THE UNKNOWN FUTURE

RETURN OF SELFESTEEM

DESIRE TO ESCAPE GOES

ADJUSTMENT TO FAMILY NEEDS

REBIRTH OF IDEALS

APPRECIATION OF REAL VALUES

FIRST STEPS TOWARDS ECONOMIC STABILITY

CARE OF PERSONAL APPEARANCE

RATIONALISATIONS RECOGNIZED

GROUP THERAPY AND MUTUAL HELP CONTINUE

CONFIDENCE OF EMPLOYERS

INCREASING TOLERANCE

CONTENTMENT IN SOBRIETY

REHABILITATION

Figure 1

Co-Dependency and its Progression

START

SYMPTOMS

OCCASIONAL RELIEF DRINKING BY ALCOHOLIC
SPOUSE HAS OCCASIONAL DOUBTS

SPOUSE RATIONALIZES ALCOHOLIC BEHAVIOR

SPOUSE ACCEPTS INCREASED DRINKING

SPOUSE INCREASINGLY DEPENDENT ON ALCOHOLIC BEHAVIOR

SPOUSE CONTROLS SURREPTITIOUSLY & SPONTANEOUSLY

SPOUSE HAS FEELINGS OF GUILT

INITIAL STAGE

SPOUSE UNABLE TO DISCUSS PROBLEM

SPOUSE DOUBTS SANITY

SPOUSE CONSTANTLY CRITICAL

SPOUSE MAKES EXCUSES TO FAMILY & FRIENDS

SPOUSE HIDES FEARS WITH GRANDIOSE & AGRESSIVE BEHAVIOR

SPOUSE EXPERIENCES SELF PITY

SPOUSE EXPERIENCES FALSE HOPE

SPOUSE'S EFFORTS TO CONTROL ALCOHOLIC FAIL

SPOUSE LOSES EMOTIONAL CONTROL

CRUCIAL PHASE

SPOUSE AWARE OF WORK & MONEY PROBLEMS

SPOUSE BECOMES OVER INVOLVED IN OUTSIDE ACTIVITIES

SPOUSE NEGLECTS FOOD

SPOUSE AVOIDS FAMILY & FRIENDS

SPOUSE SUFFERS PHYSICAL DETERIORATION

SPOUSE HAS UNREASONABLE RESENTMENTS

SPOUSE LOSES WILL POWER

SPOUSE SUFFERS MORAL DETERIORATION

SPOUSE MAKES IDLE THREATS

SPOUSE IMMOBILIZED

SPOUSE HAS IMPAIRED THINKING

SPOUSE UNABLE TO INITIATE ACTION

CHRONIC PHASE

SPOUSE HAS INDEFINABLE FEARS

SPOUSE OBSESSED WITH ALCOHOLIC DRINKING

SPOUSE HAS VAGUE SPIRITUAL DESIRES

SPOUSE EXHAUSTS ALL ALIBIS

SPOUSE ADMITS DEFEAT

SURRENDER

EDUCATION

SPOUSE ACCEPTS ALCOHOLISM AS DISEASE

SPOUSE DESIRES HELP – STARTS WITH SUPPORT GROUP (AL ANON)

SPOUSE STOPS REACTING TO ALCOHOLIC BEHAVIOR

SPOUSE TAKES PERSONAL INVENTORY

SPOUSE EXPERIENCES RENEWED HOPE

GROWTH

SPOUSE'S SELF CONFIDENCE RETURNS

SPOUSE IMPROVES PERSONAL RELATIONSHIPS

SPOUSE APPRECIATES INDEPENDENCE

SPOUSE DEVELOPS SELF ESTEEM

SPOUSE RECOGNIZES OWN NEEDS AND VALUES

SPOUSE FACES REALITY

SPOUSE WIDENS CIRCLE OF FRIENDS

SUPPORT

SPOUSE REGAINS EMOTIONAL STABILITY

SPOUSE SHARES STRENGTH WITH SUPPORT GROUP

SPOUSE CONTINUES WITH SUPPORT GROUP

RECOVERY

*CO-DEPENDENCY IS AN ILLNESS SUFFERED BY THOSE PERSONS EMOTIONALLY INVOLVED WITH AN ALCOHOLIC

Figure 2

to more than one substance. The ability of alcoholics/addicts to change their addictive use from one drug to another is seen in many settings. When drug addicts or alcoholics begin to worry about their dependence on a particular substance, they often switch to another drug, trying to convince themselves that they really aren't hooked.

Alan S., for example, had been a "recreational" drug user in his early twenties. He smoked marijuana, drank "socially," took hallucinogens such as LSD, and tried cocaine several times. His life was stable, however, as he was developing a professional career and had gotten married. He only used alcohol and drugs at parties and with friends. He certainly didn't think he had a problem.

Alan was always restless and intermittently depressed, but he put on a good act, and most people he knew regarded him as successful. One day he sustained a back injury, and his doctor prescribed Percodan for pain. Alan found the Percodan not only relieved the discomfort but also gave him a delightful feeling. He looked forward to each dose, and he took the pills for a general sense of well-being even after the pain had subsided. When the prescription ran out, he didn't seek more pills immediately, but he remembered their effect.

One night weeks later, Alan didn't sleep well, and the following day he was anxious and uncomfortable. He thought that Percodan would help relieve his discomfort, so he called his doctor, told him his back was acting up, and got a prescription for Percodan. The pills really did the trick.

For five years, Alan used Percodan periodically. At times he would become physically addicted and would put himself through painful and disruptive days of withdrawal. He felt anxious about being addicted, but thought he had just gone a bit too far. Each time he stopped the pills, a certain tension would build, and within a few weeks he'd start using them again.

During this time, Alan continued his recreational drug use as well. He smoked marijuana, used more and more cocaine, and began to take Valium and other prescription drugs. Although he believed he was just someone who liked to have a good time, periodically he worried that he was taking too many drugs. He sometimes wondered whether anxiety and depression made him use drugs and alcohol, but most of the time, he avoided thinking about it.

As he became more worried about his dependence on drugs and as the effort to obtain them became more stressful, Alan turned more and more to alcohol. Before long, his daily vodka intake approached a fifth a day. He couldn't drink at work, however, and the days became intolerably stressful. There was an internal, irritable tension he could barely stand. Soon he was back to ingesting a mixture of drugs (usually Percodan and Valium) during the day, and alcohol at night.

For several years Alan tried to control his alcohol use, only to see his drug intake increase; then he tried to control his drug use, only to find his alcohol consumption increase. His life finally consisted of periods of horrible tension and discomfort interspersed with periods of drug or alcohol-induced oblivion. He ended up in a treatment center.

Many alcoholics and addicts have stories resembling Alan's. Their disease is addiction, and any mood-altering substance will serve to keep it alive.

Cocaine addicts may believe that alcohol is not their problem, but case after case shows that cocaine addicts cannot drink alcohol if they want to arrest their disease and recover. Similarly, the alcoholic who never abused other drugs cannot, in recovery, smoke marijuana, take Valium, or snort cocaine. When recovering alcoholics and addicts try to give up their drug of choice but still use another, they stop their growth in recovery and begin an inevitable course back to their drug of choice or into uncontrollable use of the secondary substance. Interviews with AA members indicate that occasional cases like this occur in an AA group—cases in which a member smokes marijuana or abuses prescription narcotics while attending AA meetings, eventually relapsing into runaway addiction with alcohol or drugs.

Similar examples were also seen in addicts who had been through a number of the early heroin recovery programs in the 1960s and 1970s. Cross-addiction was little understood at the time, and recovering heroin addicts often left recovery programs without having been warned against alcohol. Years later many of these same people developed alcoholism and entered treatment centers, having learned the hard way that any mood-altering substance can take hold of the reins of their disease.

Dually addicted alcoholics/addicts (those who abuse two substances) usually realize the need for total abstinence in recovery. The alcoholics/addicts who have the most trouble understanding the need to avoid all mood-altering drugs are those who abused only one substance. The pure alcoholic finds it hard to accept the danger of taking codeine or Valium. Drugs, he often feels, were not his problem. Similarly, recovering cocaine addicts often find it hard to accept that they can never drink.

Nevertheless, as experience with recovering alcoholics/addicts accumulates, the principle becomes clear:

Recovering alcoholics and addicts must avoid all mood-altering substances for the rest of their lives.

If they do not, they run a very high risk of becoming active alcoholics/addicts once again. This road back to the drug of choice is not always direct, but once a mood-changing drug is allowed to trigger the disease of addiction, eventually the individual will return to uncontrollable substance abuse.

Tony M., for example, was a narcotics addict who hit bottom after developing a life-threatening infection from an unsterile injection. Tony, a lawyer, finally realized the depths to which his life had fallen. He began a drug rehabilitation program in earnest. He was deeply dedicated to recovering and, with difficulty, made solid progress. He spent three and a half years in this outpatient program. After this he did well for three more years, when a "little voice" told him he was all right and could have a little wine with dinner. That one glass of wine led, within weeks, to considerably more wine, and soon Tony was drinking the way he had formerly used heroin. After another year, he began using a prescription narcotic, and only a few weeks later he was in a detoxification ward, having lost his family and his career.

Two

Safe Medical Caregivers:

CHOOSING AND WORKING
WITH DOCTORS

Each recovering alcoholic/addict encounters the need for medical care. Sometimes the need is minor, such as treatment of a respiratory infection. Sometimes there are more significant problems requiring medical procedures or treatment; sometimes surgery is needed, and so anesthesia and pain must be considered. How can a person in recovery approach these emotionally difficult situations while maximally protecting sobriety?

As mentioned previously, it is better to anticipate the problems presented by the medical world than to find yourself plunged into the center of an anxiety-ridden medical problem without having considered your special needs as a recovering alcoholic or addict.

How do you choose a doctor? What specifics do you tell your physician? What pitfalls does medical treatment present? When undergoing surgery, why must you tell the anesthesiologist about your disease and its idiosyncrasies? How much understanding and knowledge of alcoholism and addiction can you expect from the medical world? These questions are better considered before the need arises.

Proceeding carefully when deciding on medical care is crucial for several reasons—some obvious, some more subtle. It is obvious that because drugs are prescribed by doctors, both you and the doctor must clearly understand the potential dangers carried by mind-altering or affect-changing medications.

It is less obvious that sobriety is more vulnerable when pain overtakes the recovering individual, as well as when the anxiety and fear of health-threatening conditions must be faced. Should you bear physical pain without the usual help provided by analgesic medications? Which threatens sobriety more—debilitating pain or narcotic medication? These are complex questions. There aren't always answers that are obviously right or wrong. However, the best decision can be made only by a knowledgeable physician and by the patient who has taken sobriety into account and is aware of the dangers inherent in the medical treatment.

In considering these issues, you must discuss your options with your close associates in AA. The importance of open decision making cannot be overemphasized. A recovering alcoholic or addict learns that it's essential to share decisions highly charged with emotion. The disease of alcoholism is always present to distort reasoning. Thus, it is vitally important for you *not* to plan in secret when the issues at hand can directly threaten your sobriety.

Be Sure Your Doctor Understands Alcoholism/Addiction

How do you choose a doctor who will safeguard rather than imperil sobriety? Some people already have a physician when they begin recovery, one with whom they have established a good relationship. If you have such a physician, it is important to know what understanding he or she has about the disease of alcoholism. Make an appointment with your physician and do your best to discuss the issue openly. Remember, your doctor has many other things to take into consideration, and he or she may not give the issue the same importance that you do.

Tell the doctor that you have realized you are an alcoholic (or an addict) and that you have begun your recovery. Remind the doctor you have a disease, and say you have been warned about taking certain medications. If the physician is well versed in these concepts, it should soon be apparent. If he or she is not so aware of these ideas, however, it is understandable. Although medical training in the disease of alcoholism has improved in recent years, many health-care professionals still lack clinical experience in this field.

If your doctor is open to the issue and your relationship is comfortable, you can build on this basic understanding during future encounters. On the other hand, if your doctor resists the disease concept or doesn't fully accept the dangers of mind-altering medications (pain relievers, tranquilizers, sleep medications, and so on), you should seriously consider finding another physician. An alcoholic/addict cannot take the chance of receiving medical care from a doctor who won't accept certain basic principles about recovery from addiction.

First, the physician must understand that alcoholism or addiction is a disease that is never cured, but only arrested on a daily basis. Second, the physician must also understand that drugs that affect mood (that is, drugs that sedate, that are euphoric, or that are "uppers") are potentially fatal to the recovering individual. An alcoholic/addict most often has a drug of choice. Recovery stops the compulsive behavior of using this drug. However, any mind-altering substance can either directly trigger the old compulsive behavior or indirectly weaken the state of abstinence, eventually allowing the compulsive disorder to reestablish itself. Thus it is critical for the recovering person to find a physician who understands this.

Finally, in discussions with a potential physician, take care not to mount a crusade to educate him or her. Simply assess whether the doctor understands the basic concepts necessary to protect sobriety.

Finding Doctors Who Understand the Disease

If you do not have an appropriate physician for your basic medical care, how can you find one? Word of mouth can often help. You can ask friends in AA (or similar recovery program) or call a nearby rehabilitation center for referrals. (Recovery-program friends could probably identify a treatment center or two.) You might also call the AA information number given in your area's telephone directory.

You can also locate treatment centers on-line by visiting http://findtreatment.samhsa.gov. There you will find information on more than 11,000 treatment programs, including names, addresses, and phone numbers. The site is provided by the Substance Abuse and Mental Health Services Administration (SAMHSA) of the U.S. Department of Health and Human Services.

Doctors Certified in Addiction Medicine or Addiction Psychiatry

Another way of locating a physician well informed about alcoholism/ addiction is to find one who is certified by the American Society of

Addiction Medicine (ASAM) or the American Academy of Addiction Psychiatry (AAAP). The ASAM, which began as the New York City Medical Society on Alcoholism in 1954, expanded in scope and numbers over the years, and adopted its present name in 1989. Today, ASAM is an association of some 3,700 physicians from virtually all medical specialties and subspecialties, declares an ASAM report, who are dedicated to improving the treatment of alcoholism and other addictions.

Physicians qualify for ASAM's certification in addiction medicine by meeting specified high standards in training, in experience, and on the examination for certification. Recertification by exam is required every ten years.

According to the American Academy of Addiction Psychiatry, AAAP is a professional membership organization founded in 1985 with approximately 1,000 members in the United States and around the world. Among its aims in addiction psychiatry are seeking to improve treatment, public understanding and policy, professional continuing education, and research. The group also conducts an addiction psychiatry review course that can help prepare candidates for the subspecialty certification exam in addiction psychiatry. Moreover, it provides information about such subspecialty certification, which is offered by the American Board of Psychiatry and Neurology.

One way to locate physicians qualified in treating addiction is by going to the Web site of the American Medical Association (AMA) at http://www.ama-assn.org. Near the top left of the AMA homepage is a header reading Patients. Click GO. Again, on the left, you will see Doctor Finder. Click on that. You will then see a screen enabling you to search among more than 600,000 doctors in all specialties and subspecialties. Type in the cities or towns you're interested in, and the specialties (or subspecialties) you want. You will then be provided with the names of the appropriate physicians. Note that subspecialties in both addiction medicine and addiction psychiatry are included in the AMA database.

Dangerous Areas of Medical Treatment

The areas of medical treatment most fraught with danger for recovering alcoholics/addicts are the use of anesthesia and the treatment of pain.

Mild pain caused by most headaches, muscle and joint sprains, and the like can be handled easily. Don't even consider taking dangerous drugs   that is, possibly habit-forming or addictive ones. (See Chapter 3). Perhaps no drugs at all should be used for mild pain, since it might be best to resist the reflex to take a drug for every uncomfortable situation. Try heat or ice packs, hot showers, massages, or other mechanical measures to ease minor pain. However, when such mechanical measures may not be enough, try aspirin, acetaminophen (as in Tylenol), or ibuprofen to relieve minor pain. (These and other safe analgesics, or pain relievers, are listed in Chapter 3.)

Moderate and severe pain, particularly postoperative pain, require more serious consideration. Alcoholics are often told that when medically indicated, narcotic drugs and the like can be used. However, this is not a simple matter. Everyone's pain threshhold differs, and "medically indicated" is not an absolute. The authors believe that if pain is severe, a recovering alcoholic or addict can justifiably use narcotic analgesic medications that are habit-forming (and hence normally dangerous for them). But this should be done only with certain precautions.

Any alcoholic/addict who goes into an operating room takes a dangerous disease along. Therefore he must plan carefully to protect his sobriety. The potential danger cannot be combated effectively in the state of mind that exists postoperatively, when pain and the effects of anesthesia distort thinking. Moreover, if narcotics were among the alcoholic/addict's drugs of choice, then he or she is all the more vulnerable. Advance planning is thus essential.

If you are anticipating pain from a surgical procedure, discuss your plans for postoperative pain medication with your sponsor in AA (or similar recovery program) and with other friends in the program. As mentioned, it is dangerous for you to make these decisions alone. If you keep your plans secret, your addiction-prone mind will almost surely find rationalizations to take drugs inappropriately or will fall into one of numerous traps that the compulsive disease offers.

Coping with Severe Pain

The authors consider the following instructions essential for getting through postoperative or other severe pain with maximum safety.

1. Discuss the situation, and design a plan before surgery, as described previously.
2. Discuss the plan with the doctor beforehand.
3. Keep a written log of all pain medications and sedatives you take. Doing this prevents distortions and self-deception about the amount of medication used. Review this log with your sponsor or friends in your recovery program.
4. Stop using the pain medication as soon as possible. First, discontinue injections at the earliest feasible time, and then discontinue pills—preferably before going home from the hospital. Enduring some pain may be the price you have to pay.

5. If treatment includes the continued use of pain pills at home, continue to maintain a written log of the number and frequency of pills taken.

6. Preferably, give the pills to a close friend in your recovery program to administer when they are needed. Having to ask for them will keep you honest.

7. Once treatment ends, discard all unused medications immediately.

Coping with Surgery and Anesthesia

An alcoholic/addict who faces surgery must take special care with regard to anesthesia. Discuss your situation with the anesthesiologist as well as the surgeon. Tell the doctors which classes or types of drugs you have abused. Be clear about your drugs of choice. If tranquilizers, sedatives, or narcotics must be administered during your hospitalization, then ask whether the drugs used could be of a different class from your drugs of choice. This is important because, although any mood-changing substance carries a certain risk, the authors believe that using a drug of choice carries the danger of triggering the as yet unexplained physiologic or psychologic reflexes of addiction. If nothing else, the experience of "getting high" with a drug of choice will bring with it all the feelings and memories of your days of abuse. However, even if alcohol was your only drug of choice, don't forget that the basic principle still holds: any mood-changing medication (sedatives, narcotics, and so on) is dangerous for you.

In interviewing numerous recovering persons, the authors have found that many medications elicit unexpected or idiosyncratic responses in the alcoholic or addict. Whether you have abused alcohol, other drugs, or both, you need to anticipate possible unpredictable responses to pain relievers, anesthetics, sedatives, and even everyday drugs such as decongestants.

For example, many alcoholics report requiring much heavier than normal doses of pain medication postoperatively or in other painful circumstances (such as dental pain or bone fractures). On the other hand, many alcoholics and narcotics addicts report being overly reactive to pain medications—that is, they require lower than normal doses, and have actually overdosed on normal amounts. The exact response to a medication cannot be predicted, but some unusual reaction should be anticipated.

Discuss these principles with your doctors. The anesthesiologist in particular should be warned to expect unusual reactions to medications. This warning can be invaluable for the optimal and safe anesthetic administration and care.

In summary, before any major surgery, as an alcoholic/addict, you must reach an understanding with your doctor and anesthesiologist by clearly conveying and emphasizing the following points.

1. Your former drug or drugs of choice should be avoided, if at all possible.
2. Any mood-changing substances carry cross-addiction potential for you and generally have a risk of triggering dangerous mechanisms of addiction.
3. You may exhibit unusual reactions to various medications.

Three

Safe—and Highly Unsafe— Medicines in Recovery:

A COMPREHENSIVE DIRECTORY

Medications present recovering alcoholics and addicts with special and crucial risks. Many medications—including certain pain relievers, sedatives, and cough remedies—contain ingredients that may be habit-forming. Such substances are only possibly addictive for nonalcoholics and nonaddicts, but they have caused recurrences of active alcoholism and addiction in substantial numbers of recovering individuals. Thus alcoholics and addicts must be aware that these addictive medications can be highly dangerous, even lethal. For maximum protection against their hazards, a recovering alcoholic addict should carry out the following key actions when planning to use—or when using—any medications.

1. Be honest and frank with your doctors and your sponsor.
2. Use alternatives to pills to help break a "pills habit."
3. Discard hazardous medications as soon as the period of legitimate use ends.

4. Watch out for lies you tell doctors in order to obtain medications.
5. Watch out for lies you tell yourself in order to justify getting medications.

This chapter explains why each of these five actions is vital and how to carry them out. It also provides an extensive list of medications; with it, you can assess the danger or safety of many hundreds of the most common medications when used by recovering alcoholics/addicts.

Why Medications Endanger Recovering Alcoholics/Addicts

The principle of cross-addiction (see Chapter 1) demonstrates that exposure to any mood-altering substance can trigger the pathology of addiction. Alcohol or specifically abused drugs need not be the trigger. Rather, any substance with addictive potential or mood-altering properties can lower one's resistance to the compulsive use of alcohol or drugs. Such substances trigger in the recovering alcoholic/addict a cascade of events that often ends in the revival of addiction—usually in an even more acute and terrifying form than before.

By no means does the alcoholic/addict have a simple reaction consisting merely of a euphoric "high" followed by the loss of willpower and control. Rather, ingestion of a potentially addictive substance sets off a whole series of events accompanied by lowered resistance to the latent disease of alcoholism/addiction. Individuals appear to vary in the extent to which their resistance is lowered, but risk develops with any drop in resistance.

How to Guard against Dangers from Medicines

BE HONEST WITH DOCTORS AND YOUR SPONSOR

When confronted with the possible need for medication, it is important that the alcoholic/addict suspend his or her own judgment, and instead rely on those who are more familiar with the disease of alcoholism/addiction. These include one's sponsor or experienced guide in AA or other recovery program, as well as physicians who are knowledgeable about the disease. With such advisers, the alcoholic/addict should be truthful and frank about every aspect of any need for medication, including pain, distress, and past reactions to medications.

USE ALTERNATIVES TO PILLS TO HELP BREAK A "PILLS HABIT"

Alcoholics/addicts starting in recovery programs often have a habit of taking pills to treat every health problem. "Pill seeking behavior" is the professional term for this habit. They are usually advised to substitute new measures to relieving conditions that have been occasions for pill-taking. For example, individuals considering using aspirin for a mild headache may be told to take a cold shower instead.

A summary of minor health problems and some ways to relieve them without taking pills follows. Of course, if any of your symptoms are severe, consult your physician.

Health Problem	How to Relieve without Taking Pills
Headache	Have a shower (perhaps a cold one).
Sleeplessness	Take a warm bath; drink warm milk; read recovery literature; get daytime exercise to relax the body physically.
Constipation	Eat prunes or drink prune juice; eat or drink other fruits or fruit juices; drink eight to ten large glasses of water daily.
Anxiety, tension	Breathe slowly and deeply for 5 minutes at a stretch; practice relaxation techniques.
Drowsiness	Stretch; exercise; drink tea or coffee; practice vigorous deep breathing; sleep as appropriate.
Diarrhea	Drink a lot of fluids; eat no fresh fruits; be patient.
Depression	Do enjoyable exercise; perform useful manual tasks; phone or meet with sponsor or other recovery-program friend.

DISCARD HAZARDOUS MEDICATION

Individuals recovering from substance abuse are commonly advised to dispose of any potentially dangerous medication as soon as the time for which it was prescribed has ended. Doing so helps prevent later addictive abuse of the medication.

How important it is to take this precaution is illustrated by the case of Tina M. A middle-aged attorney, Tina suffered whiplash in an auto accident. She didn't tell her doctor that she was a recovering alcoholic. As a result, the doctor prescribed Talwin, a potentially habit-forming analgesic, to relieve recurrent headaches caused by the injury. He told Tina to use the medication no longer than a week. Within four days her headaches ended, and Tina stopped taking the Talwin. But she left the bottle containing several unused tablets in her medicine chest.

Six months later, Tina lost an important case, and her son broke his leg in an accident that wrecked the family's best car. She began to feel utterly hopeless, and one morning she noticed the Talwin bottle while putting on her makeup. Almost by reflex she reached out and took two tablets. She soon felt much better. That night she drank a little cognac after dinner to help her unwind. Within three weeks she started on the worst binge of her life, and a week later she entered an alcoholism treatment center.

WATCH OUT FOR LIES YOU TELL DOCTORS

Their compulsions often lead alcoholics/addicts to distort the truth with doctors in order to get medications they consider imperative for relief. Any imaginable untruth may be told to the doctor with a sense of complete justification by the alcoholic/addict. He or she may lie about the intensity of pain or other discomfort, and he may even pretend to have pain when none is present.

Recovering alcoholics/addicts sometimes con doctors just as unconsciously as do those who are actively practicing their addictions. As a result, it is recommended that the recovering alcoholic/addict be completely up-front with his or her sponsor about all plans to obtain medications; the alcoholic/addict must also be on guard against a possible predisposition to mislead doctors. Of course, doctors are urged to be on the alert for such tendencies and to avoid being taken in by them

WATCH OUT FOR LIES YOU TELL YOURSELF

Conning a doctor in order to obtain unnecessary or even hazardous medications is often done by alcoholics/addicts in all sincerity. In such instances, their disease of addiction first misleads them, and they then need feel no restraint in saying whatever may work in fooling the doctor.

Accordingly, recovering alcoholics/addicts must understand that such self-deception is likely, and they should discount their own convictions on questions of medications. Being completely honest with one's sponsor and other advisers in recovery programs helps prevent such self-deception.

Hazards—or Safety—of Medications by Type

This section provides a unique guide to the dangers or safety for sobriety of hundreds of medications. The section covers both prescription and nonprescription medications. Types of medications are presented in alphabetical order of the type names. Under the type name appears essential information about the potential danger or safety for alcoholics/adults of medications of this type. After this information, each medication of that type is listed by trade name and generic name (in alphabetical order). Medications of each type are presented in catagories grouped as follows:

UNSAFE: medications that pose potential danger (that is, high risk) of relapse into alcoholism/addiction by recovering alcoholics/addicts.

SAFE: medications that are safe (that is, without risk) with respect to continued abstinence.

CHANCY: medications that might pose a risk of reactivating full-blown alcoholism/addiction—unless used with certain specified precautions.

Types of medications listed here are identified by type, such as "Antihypertensive Agents (High Blood Pressure Medications)" or "Hormones." Text after the type-name heading identifies drugs of this type as unsafe, safe, or chancy; briefly indicates their major uses; and names a few widely used drugs of this type as illustrative examples.

Use this section to find out about the potential dangers—or safety of medication as follows:

1. Use the index at the back of the book to locate the page number for a particular medication.
2. Turn to the appropriate page, and find the listing for the medication. Note any special advice that may be given right after the medication's name.
3. Then move back to the information presented at the start of the type under which the medication is listed, and consult that information.

Note: If you cannot find a medication in the index, do the following:

1. Look up the name of the *type* of medication instead. (You can find out the type from your doctor or pharmacist, if you don't already know it.)
2. Turn to the page number given for that type of medication, and read the information appearing after the type name.
3. If any medication—or type of medication—on which you seek advice is not listed, do not use the medication until you

have consulted a doctor well informed on alcoholism/ addiction about its possible hazards or safety.

The section covers the following major types of medications, in the following order:

Medications That Call for Special Caution (lists individual medications)

Analgesics That Are Narcotics or Controlled Substances (lists individual medications)

Analgesics (Pain Relievers), Antipyretics (Antifever Drugs), and Antimigraine Agents That Are Not Narcotics or Addictive Controlled Substances (lists individual medications)

Anesthetics (lists individual medications)

Antiallergy Medications (Antihistamines/Antipruritics [anti-itching drugs]/Mast-Cell Stabilizers) (lists individual medications)

Antiarthritic Agents

Antiasthmatics (Bronchodilators)

Antibiotics

Anticancer Agents (Antineoplastics)

Anticoagulants

Anticonvulsants (lists individual medications)

Antidiabetics (Hypoglycemic Agents)

Antidyskinetics (relieve involuntary shaking or tremors) (Antiparkinsonism Agents)

Antifungal Agents; Antiviral Agents

Antigout Agents

Antihypertensive Agents (High Blood Pressure Medications)

Antiplatelet Agents (prevent blood clots)

Corticosteroids (hormones made by the adrenal glands) (lists
   individual medications)

Cough, Cold, or Other Upper Respiratory Medications (lists
   individual medications)

Dental Preparations (lists individual medications)

Diagnostics

Diuretics ("Water Pills")

Gastrointestinal System Medications:

   Antacids, Antiflatulents, Digestants

   Antidiarrheal Agents; Oral Electrolyte Solutions (lists indi-
      vidual medications)

   Antinauseants (Antiemetics, Anti-Motion Sickness Agents),
      (lists individual medications)

   Antiulcer-Antisecretory Agents; Antispasmodics

   Laxatives; Stool Softeners (lists individual medications)

Geriatric Medications

Heart Disease Medications

Hemorrhoidal Medications

HIV/AIDS Medications

Hormones

Muscle Relaxants (lists individual medications)

Parasitic Disease Medications

Potassium Supplements

Psychotherapeutic Agents (lists individual medications):

   Antianxiety Agents (Minor Tranquilizers)

   Antidepressants

   Major Tranquilizers (Antipsychotics)

   Central Nervous System (CNS) Stimulants

Sedatives/Hypnotics (lists individual medications)

Serum Cholesterol-Lowering and Fat-Lowering Medications
   (Hypolipidemics) (used in treating heart conditions)

Smoking Cessation Medications

Urinary Tract Agents

Vitamin and Mineral Supplements; Nutritionals

Contraceptives

Important Note: UNSAFE and SAFE, when attributed to an individual medication or type of medication in this book, indicate only the following:

First, these terms apply only to use of the medication (or medication type) by men and women recovering from alcohol or drug abuse.

Second, these terms apply only to the possible effect of taking that medication (or medication type) on continued abstinence from substance abuse by such recovering persons. That is, the word UNSAFE is employed to indicate that taking the medication may tend to reactivate the person's substance abuse; the word SAFE indicates that taking the medication will probably not tend to reactivate the person's substance abuse.

Attributions of these terms in these specific senses are based on information about the medications provided to the public by the producers of the medications and supplemented by widespread clinical experience and practice, as well as by the experience of those in the field of alcoholism and drug addiction. (That information about a medication provided to the public concerns such effects as action as a central nervous system depressant, tendency to be habit-forming, tendency to induce a mood of euphoria, tendency to relieve a mood of depression, and tendency to induce drowsiness or sleep.)

Third, characterization in this chapter as SAFE or UNSAFE as defined here is provided only for general information. It is not set forth as either medical counseling or medical treatment. Readers should take (or should not take) any medications—including those referred to in this book—only as advised by their physicians.

In addition, all names of medications presented in this chapter (and throughout the book) with the initial letter (or letters) of their names capitalized are trade names or registered trademarks of their producers and/or distributors.

Essential Reference Listing of Each Medication's Dangers or Safety for Recovering Alcoholics/Addicts

Names of medications most often shown in the listing are brand names. Medications or drugs are also shown in the listing by their generic name (scientific, chemical, or other established-usage name that is not a registered trademark). In some cases, medications are also shown by their street names—that is, names given them in conversational usage such as "uppers," "downers," or "diet pills."

Typographic style used in the listing to indicate the type of name being given is as follows (such style parallels conventional practice):

Trade Name: given in initial capital (or uppercase) letters, for example, Anaprox-DS Tablets

generic name: given in lowercase letters, for example, codeine

"street name": given in lowercase letters and enclosed in double quotation marks, for example, "downers"

After each brand (or street name), the chemical or generic names of the major active ingredients in that drug are given.

For each type of medication, up to four subcategories are presented, in the following order:

Prescription Drugs that Are UNSAFE

Prescription Drugs that Are SAFE

Nonprescription Drugs that Are UNSAFE

Nonprescription Drugs that Are SAFE

Medications That Are HIGHLY UNSAFE

Recovering alcoholics/addicts should make every effort to avoid taking the medications in this section. These medications have particularly euphoric effects—to such an extent that the way in which they act in the system may even extend beyond our present understanding.

Many an addictive career has been started by the prescribing of these medications for legitimate medical problems. In addition, many actively addicted individuals drift toward abuse of these medications.

Individuals recovering from substance abuse either should not take any of these or should observe every possible precaution while using one if it has been recommended as essential by a doctor thoroughly informed about alcoholism/addiction. Alternatives and precautions applicable to the following medications, most of which are used to relieve acute pain, are set forth in the section "Pain" in Chapter 4. And as an example, alternative cough medicines to ones like Tussionex can be found later in this chapter in "Cough, Cold, or Other Upper-Respiratory Medications."

The following medications call for very special caution by recovering alcoholics/addicts.

Demerol
Dilaudid
Hycodan
Hydrocet
hydrocodone (often in the form hydrocodone bitartrate)
hydromorphone (often in the form hydromorphone hydro-
    chloride)
Hy-Phen (formerly Hycodaphen)

Levo-Dromoran
levorphanol (often in the form levorphanol tartrate)
meperidene (often in the form meperidene hydrochloride)
oxycodone
OxyContin
Percocet
Percodan
Roxicodone
SK-Oxycodone
Tussionex Pennkinetic (cough suppressant and antihistamine)
Tylox
Vicodin
Zydone

Analgesics: Narcotics or Controlled Substances UNSAFE

Narcotics, addictive drugs that produce physical and psychological dependence in the user, were first nationally regulated in the United States under the Harrison Narcotics Tax Act of 1914. Narcotics include opium and its derivatives (heroin, morphine, and codeine), as well as synthetic drugs, such as meperidine and methadone, that can bring about morphinelike addiction. In addition, some state laws define cocaine and marijuana as narcotics.

Drugs that have been widely abused (including nonnarcotics) are now regulated under a federal law popularly called the Controlled Substances Act (officially, Title II of the Comprehensive Drug Abuse Prevention and Control Act of 1970, Public Law 91-513). Provisions of the act are enforced by the Drug Enforcement Administration of the U.S. Department of Justice.

ADDICTION RISKS

Under the Controlled Substances Act, drugs are classified as controlled substances within its Schedules I, II, III, IV, or V. Schedule I drugs pose the highest addiction risk; drugs in Schedules II through V pose successively lesser degrees of risk. Schedule I drugs, for instance, are characterized by high potential for abuse, no accepted medical use in the United States, and no accepted medical practices for assuring safe use in the United States. Similarly, Schedule II drugs are marked by high potential for abuse, an accepted medical use in the United States (often with severe restrictions), and severe psychological or physical dependence resulting from abuse.

All the medications in this section are controlled substances. (Codeine phosphate, for example, is in Schedule II, and propoxyphene is in Schedule IV; such classifications are indicated by notations in pharmaceutical listings like "C-II" and "C-IV.") Their major medical use is to relieve unusually severe to extreme pain, and so they are most often classified as analgesics (pain relievers). They are available only by prescription.

All controlled substances are, of course, **UNSAFE** for recovering alcoholics/addicts, since they are extremely to very substantially habit-forming. A recovering alcoholic/addict should avoid them whenever possible in order to avoid the high risk of reactivating acute substance abuse.

PRECAUTIONS

Only imperative medical need should cause an individual in recovery to use a controlled substance, and, if one must be taken, the precautions stated elsewhere in this book should be taken. (See the beginning of this chapter and "Pain" in Chapter 4.) One exception applies to heroin addicts recovering in legal and strictly supervised methadone maintenance programs. In these programs, specially dispensed doses of methadone end their heroin cravings without producing euphoria.

Many controlled substances are combinations of chemicals and include nonaddictive mild pain relievers or stimulants, such as aspirin, acetaminophen, or caffeine.

The addictive or habit-forming ingredients in these medications include codeine or codeine compounds; opium; barbiturates such as pentobarbital and butalbital; oxycodone compounds; oxymorphone compounds; hydrocodone compounds; hydromorphone compounds; morphine or morphine compounds; methadone compounds; and compounds of levorphanol, alphaprodine, fentanyl, propoxyphene, meperidine, meprobamate, and pentazocine.

Acetaco Tablets
   (codeine phosphate, acetaminophen)
Acetaminophen and Codeine Phosphate Oral Solution USP, Tablets
   (codeine phosphate, acetaminophen)
Actiq
   (fentanyl citrate)
Amacodone Tablets
   (hydrocodone bitartrate, acetaminophen)
Anacin with Codeine
   (acetaminophen, codeine phosphate)
Anaplex HD Cough Syrup
   (hydrocodone bitartrate, pseudoephedrine, brompheniramine maleate)
Anexsia with Codeine
   (codeine phosphate, aspirin, caffeine)

Anexsia-D
(hydrocodone bitartrate, aspirin, caffeine)

Anolor, Anolor-300 Capsules
(butalbital, acetaminophen, caffeine)

ASA and Codeine Compound
(codeine phosphate, aspirin, caffeine)

Ascriptin with Codeine
(codeine phosphate, aspirin, magnesium-aluminum hydroxide)

Astramorph PF Injection
(morphine sulfate)

Axocet Capsules
(butalbital, acetaminophen)

Bancap-HC Capsules
(hydrocodone bitartrate, acetaminophen)

Bayapap with Codeine Elixir
(codeine phosphate, acetaminophen)

Bexophene Capsules
(propoxyphene hydrochloride, aspirin, caffeine)

B&O Supprettes
(opium, belladonna)

Bupap Tablets
(butalbital, acetaminophen)

Buprenex Injectable
(bupenorphine hydrochloride)

butalbital, aspirin, and codeine phosphate capsules

Cafergot P-B (antimigraine agent)
(pentobarbital, ergotamine tartrate, caffeine, belladonna alkaloids)

Capital with Codeine Tablets, Oral Suspension
(codeine phosphate, acetaminophen)

Cocaine Hydrochloride Topical Solution (4% or 10%)
(cocaine hydrochloride)

Codap Tablets

(codeine phosphate, acetaminophen)

codeine phosphate

Codeine Phosphate in Tubex Injection; Oral Solution

(codeine phosphate)

codeine sulfate

Codoxy

(oxycodone hydrochloride, oxycodone terephthalate, aspirin)

Co-gesic Tablets

(hydrocodone bitartrate, acetaminophen)

Damacet-P

(hydrocodone bitartrate, acetaminophen)

Damason-P

(hydrocodone bitartrate, aspirin, caffeine)

Darvocet-N 50, and Darvocet-N 100 Tablets

(propoxyphene napsylate, acetaminophen)

Darvon Compound-65 Pulvules

(propoxyphene hydrochloride, aspirin, caffeine)

Darvon Pulvules

(propoxyphene hydrochloride)

Darvon with ASA

(propoxyphene hydrochloride, aspirin)

Darvon-N Tablets

(propoxyphene napsylate)

Darvon-N with ASA

(propoxyphene napsylate, aspirin)

Demerol Tablets, Syrup

(meperidine hydrochloride)

Demerol-APAP

(meperidine hydrochloride, acetaminophen)

Dia-Gesic

(hydrocodone bitartrate, aspirin, acetaminophen, caffeine)

Dicodid
(hydrocodone)

dihydromorphinone hydrochloride
(hydromorphone)

Dilaudid Ampules, Injection, Multiple Dose, Oral Liquid, Powder, Suppositories, Tablets
(hydromorphone hydrochloride)

Dilaudid-HP Injection, Lyophilized Powder
(hydromorphone hydrochloride)

Dolacet Capsules
(hydrocodone bitartrate, acetaminophen)

Dolene Capsules
(propoxyphene hydrochloride)

Dolene AP-65 Capsules
(propoxyphene hydrochloride, acetaminophen)

Dolene Compound-65 Capsules
(propoxyphene hydrochloride, aspirin, caffeine)

Dolo-Pap
(hydrocodone bitartrate, acetaminophen)

Dolophine Hydrochloride Ampules, Vials, Tablets
(methadone hydrochloride)

Doxaphene Compound
(propoxyphene hydrochloride, aspirin, caffeine)

Duradyne DHC
(hydrocodone bitartrate, acetaminophen)

Duragesic Transdermal System
(fentanyl)

Duramorph Injection
(morphine sulfate)

Duramorph PF
(morphine)

Duratuss HD Elixir
 (hydrocodone bitartrate, pseudoephedrine, guaifenesin)
Emcodeine Tablets
 (codeine phosphate, aspirin)
Empirin with Codeine
 (aspirin, codeine phosphate)
Empracet with Codeine Phosphate
 (acetaminophen, codeine phosphate)
Endocet Tablets
 (oxycodone hydrochloride, acetominophen)
Endodan Tablets
 (oxycodone hydrochloride)
Equagesic Tablets
 (meprobamate, aspirin)
Esgic Capsules, Tablets; Esgic-Plus Tablets
 (butalbital, caffeine, acetaminophen)
Fentanyl Citrate Injection
 (fentanyl)
Fiorinal
 (butalbital, aspirin, caffeine)
Fiorinal with Codeine Capsules (often prescribed for migraine headaches)
 (butalbital, aspirin, caffeine, codeine)
Fiortal Capsules
 (butalbital)
Fiortal with Codeine Capsules
 (butalbital, codeine phosphate)
Guaifenesin Syrup with Codeine
 (codeine phosphate, guaifenesin)
Halotussin-AC Syrup
 (codeine phosphate, guaifenesin)

Halotussin-DAC Syrup
(codeine phosphate, guaifenesin, pseudoephedrine)

Hycodan Syrup, Tablets
(hydrocodone bitartrate, homatropine methylbromide)

Hycomine Compound Tablets
(hydrocodone bitartrate, chlorpheniramine maleate, phenyle-phrine hydrochloride, acetaminophen, caffeine)

Hycotuss Expectorant Syrup
(hydrocodone bitartrate, guaifenesin)

Hydrocet Capsules
(hydrocodone bitartrate, acetaminophen)

hydrocodone bitartrate with acetaminophen tablets (and in combination with other ingredients)

Hydrogesic Capsules
(hydrocodone bitartrate, acetaminophen)

hydromorphone hydrochloride

Hydromorphone Hydrochloride in Tubex, Injection, Tablets
(hydromorphone hydrochloride)

Hydropane Syrup
(hydrocodone bitartrate, homatropine methylbromide)

Hy-Phen Tablets (formerly Hycodaphen)
(hydrocodone bitartrate, acetaminophen)

Infumorph 200 Sterile Solution, Infumorph 500 Sterile Solution
(morphine sulfate)

Kadian Capsules
(morphine sulfate)

Levo-Dromoran
(levorphanol tartrate)

levorphanol tartrate tablets

Lorcet

(propoxyphene hydrochloride, acetaminophen)

Lorcet-HD Capsules, Lorcet 10/650 Tablets, Lorcet Plus Tablets

(hydrocodone bitartrate, acetaminophen)

Lortab ASA

(hydrocodone bitartrate, aspirin)

Lortab Elixir; Lortab 2.5/500, 5/500, 7.5/500, and 10/500 Tablets

(hydrocodone bitartrate, acetaminophen)

Maxidone Tablets

(hydrocodone bitartrate, acetaminophen)

Mepergan Injection; Mepergan in Tubex

(meperidine hydrochloride, promethazine hydrochloride)

meperidine hydrochloride tablets, syrup, injection

meprobamate tablets

methadone hydrochloride tablets, diskets

Methadone Hydrochloride Intensol Oral Concentrate, Oral Solution

(methadone hydrochloride)

methadone hydrochloride oral concentrate, oral solution

(methadone hydrochloride)

Methadose Dispersible Tablets; Oral Tablets

(methadone hydrochloride)

Micrainin

(meprobamate, aspirin)

Miltown Tablets

(meprobamate)

morphine sulfate injection, oral solution, tablets

Morphine Sulfate in Tubex

(morphine sulfate)

MS Contin Tablets
  (morphine sulfate)
MSIR Oral Capsules, Tablets, Oral Solution, Oral Solution Concentrate
  (morphine sulfate)
Nembutal Sodium Solution
  (pentobarbital sodium)
Nisentil
  (alphaprodine hydrochloride)
Norcet
  (hydrocodone bitartrate, acetaminophen)
Norco 5/325, 7.5/325, and 10/325 Tablets
  (hydrocodone bitartrate, acetaminophen)
Numorphan Suppositories, Injection
  (oxymorphone hydrochloride)
Oramorph SR Tablets
  (morphine sulfate)
OxyContin Tablets
  (oxycodone hydrochloride)
oxycodone hydrochloride, oxycodone terephthalate tablets (sometimes with aspirin or acetaminophen)
OxyFast Oral Concentrate Solution
  (oxycodone hydrochloride)
OxyIR Oral Capsules
  (oxycodone hydrochloride)
Panadol with Codeine
  (acetaminophen, codeine phosphate)
Pantopon
  (opium)
pentobarbital
Pentobarbital Sodium in Tubex
  (pentobarbital)

Percocet

(oxycodone hydrochloride, acetaminophen)

Percodan Tablets, Percodan-Demi

(oxycodone hydrochloride, oxycodone terephthalate, aspirin)

Percolone Tablets

(oxycodone hydrochloride)

Pentazocine and Naloxone Hydrochloride Tablets

(pentazocine hydrochloride, naloxone hydrochloride)

Pentazocine and Acetaminophen Tablets

(pentazocine hydrochloride, acetaminophen)

Pethadol

(meperidine hydrochloride)

Pethidine

(meperidine hydrochloride)

Phenaphen with Codeine Capsules

(acetaminophen, codeine phosphate)

Phenaphen-650 with Codeine

(acetaminophen, codeine phosphate)

Phenergan with Codeine Syrup

(codeine phosphate, promethazine hydrochloride, 7% alcohol)

Phrenilin Tablets, Phrenilin Forte Capsules

(butalbital, acetaminophen)

Pneumotussin 2.5 Cough Syrup, Tablets

(hydrocodone bitartrate)

Profene

(propoxyphene)

promethazine hydrochloride and codeine phosphate syrup

propoxyphene hydrochloride capsules (and in combinations with acetaminophen or aspirin)

propoxyphene napsylate and acetaminophen tablets

Protuss Liquid

(hydrocodone bitartrate, potassium guaiacolsulfonate)

Protuss-D Liquid

(hydrocodone bitartrate, potassium guaiacolsulfonate, pseudo-ephedrine)

Proval #3 Capsules

(codeine phosphate, acetaminophen)

RMS (suppositories)

(morphine sulfate)

Robitussin A-C Syrup

(codeine phosphate, guaifenesin, 3.5% alcohol)

Robitussin-DAC Syrup

(codeine phosphate, guaifenesin, pseudoephedrine, 1.9% alcohol)

Roxanol T Oral Solution; Roxanol 100 Concentrated Oral Solution, Roxanol Concentrated Oral Solution

(morphine sulfate)

Roxicet Caplets, Oral Solution, Tablets

(oxycodone hydrochloride, acetaminophen)

Roxicodone Tablets, Oral Solution; Roxicodone Intensol Oral Solution

(oxycodone hydrochloride)

Sedapap Tablets

(butalbital, acetaminophen)

SK-APAP with Codeine

(codeine phosphate, acetaminophen)

SK-65 Capsules

(propoxyphene hydrochloride)

SK-65 APAP Tablets

(propoxyphene hydrochloride, acetaminophen)

SK-65 Compound Capsules

(propoxyphene hydrochloride, aspirin, caffeine)

SK-Oxycodone

(oxycodone hydrochloride or oxycodone terephthalate, with acetaminophen or aspirin)

Soma Compound with Codeine Tablets

(codeine phosphate, aspirin, carisoprodol)

Sublimaze

(fentanyl)

Synalgos-DC

(dihydrocodeine bitartrate, aspirin, caffeine)

Talacen Caplets

(pentazocine hydrochloride, acetaminophen)

Talwin Compound

(pentazocine hydrochloride, aspirin)

Talwin Injection

(pentazocine lactate)

Talwin NX Tablets

(pentazocine hydrochloride, naloxone hydrochloride)

T-Gesic Forte

(hydrocodone bitartrate, acetaminophen)

Tussafed-HCG Syrup

(hydrocodone bitartrate, phenylephrine hydrochloride, guaifenesin)

Tussi-Organidin NR Liquid, Tussi-Organidin SNR Liquid

(codeine phosphate, guaifenesin)

Tylenol with Codeine Tablets

(codeine phosphate, acetaminophen)

Tylenol with Codeine Elixir

(codeine phosphate, acetaminophen, 7% alcohol)

Tylox Capsules

(oxycodone hydrochloride, oxycodone terephthalate, acetaminophen)

Ty-Tabs

(codeine phosphate, acetaminophen)

Vicodin-ES Tablets, Vicodin-HP Tablets

(hydrocodone bitartrate, acetaminophen)

Vicodin Tuss Expectorant
(hydrocodone bitartrate, guaifenesin)
Vicoprofen Tablets
(hydrocodone bitartrate, ibuprofen)
Wygesic
(propoxyphene hydrochloride, acetaminophen)
Zebutal Caplets
(butalbital, acetaminophen, caffeine)
Zydone Tablets
(hydrocodone bitartrate, acetaminophen)

Analgesics-Antipyretics and Antimigraine Agents: Nonnarcotics

ANALGESICS-ANTIPYRETICS: PRESCRIPTION CHANCY

Recovering alcoholics/addicts should use these prescription analgesic-antipyretics only if necessary—and then with special care. These medications have some mood-altering properties, according to their manufacturers, even though they are nonnarcotic and less euphoric in their effects than narcotics are. As a result, use of these agents could possibly reactivate acute substance abuse.

The following medications are used primarily as analgesics (pain relievers).

butorphanol tartrate
nalbuphine hydrochloride
Nubain
(nalbuphine hydrochloride)

Stadol
(butorphanol tartrate)

ANALGESICS-ANTIPYRETICS AND ANTIMIGRAINE AGENTS: PRESCRIPTION **SAFE**

In general, these analgesics-antipyretics and antimigraine agents are without reactivation risk for recovering alcoholics/addicts when used exactly as prescribed. The only (or major) active ingredient in these medications is an analgesic-antipyretic (to relieve pain and reduce fever). This and any other ingredients are not habit-forming for non-alcoholics, and hence they also tend to be **SAFE** for alcoholics.

ANALGESICS-ANTIPYRETICS

Anaprox Tablets, Anaprox DS Tablets
(naproxen sodium)

Diflunisal Tablets
(diflunisal)

Dolobid
(diflunisal)

Levoprome
(methotrimeprazine)

Magan
(magnesium salicylate)

Motrin
(ibuprofen)

Nalfon
(fenoprofen calcium)

Ponstel
(mefenamic acid)

Rufen
(ibuprofen)

sodium salicylate
sodium thiosalicylate

ANTIMIGRAINE AGENTS

Amerge Tablets
  (naratriptan hydrochloride)

Axert Tablets
  (timolol maleate)

Cafergot
  (ergotamine tartrate, caffeine)

Depakote Tablets
  (divalprox sodium)

D.H.E. 45 Injection
  (dihydroergotamine mesylate)

Imitrex Injection, Nasal Spray, Tablets
  (sumatriptan succinate)

**Inderal Injectable, Tablets; Inderal LA Long-Acting
  Capsules**
  (propanolol hydrochloride)

Maxalt Tablets
  (rizatriptan benzoate)

Midrin Capsules
  (isometheptene mucate, dichloralphenazone, acetaminophen)

Migranol Nasal Spray
  (dihydroergotamine mesylate)

Sansert
  (methysergide maleate)

Wigraine
  (ergotamine tartrate, caffeine)

Zomig Tablets, Zomig-ZMT Tablets
  (zolmitriptan)

ANALGESICS-ANTIPYRETICS: NONPRESCRIPTION **UNSAFE**

Nonprescription analgesics-antipyretics and similar liquid medicines used to relieve pain and/or reduce fever pose a risk for recovering alcoholics/addicts—but unfortunately it is one that is easily overlooked. The danger stems from inclusion of alcohol in the liquid medium used for many of these medications. And any alcohol intake whatsoever can bring a high reactivation risk to a recovering person.

Avoid these medications and any others containing alcohol. With any over-the-counter liquid medication, check the label and pass up those that have any alcohol content. (For pain-relief/fever-relief medications, you can easily substitute a nonliquid form containing no alcohol.) Finally, when any liquid medication is prescribed for you, ask your doctor to specify a no-alcohol-content form and then confirm with your pharmacist that the substance is alcohol-free.

Peedee Dose Aspirin Alternative
(10% alcohol, acetaminophen)

St. Joseph Aspirin-Free Elixir (7% alcohol), Infant Drops (10% alcohol)
(alcohol, acetaminophen)

ANALGESICS-ANTIPYRETICS: NONPRESCRIPTION **SAFE**

In general, nonprescription analgesics-antipyretics are without reactivation risk for recovering alcoholics/addicts when used exactly as prescribed. The only (or major) active ingredient in these medications is an analgesic-antipyretic (to relieve pain and/or reduce fever). This and any other ingredients are not habit-forming for nonalcoholics, and hence they also tend to be **SAFE** for recovering alcoholics/addicts.

The prime active ingredient in these medications is typically aspirin or acetaminophen, neither of which is habit-forming. However, some strongly addiction-prone individuals have abused aspirin or acetaminophen by taking it (often in unwisely large quantities) over long periods when its use was not justified by their pain. This is an example of addictive behavior with a substance that is not in itself habit-forming.

acetaminophen
Advil: **Advil Caplets, Gelcaps, Liquid-Gels, Tablets; Children's Advil Oral Suspension, Chewable Tablets; Infants' Advil Concentrated Drops; Junior Strength Advil Tablets, Chewable Tablets; Advil Migraine Liquigels**
   (ibuprofen)
Aleve Caplets, Gelcaps, Tablets
   (naproxen sodium)
Alka-Seltzer Antacid and Pain Reliever Effervescent Tablets (Original, Cherry, Lemon-Lime)
   (aspirin, sodium bicarbonate, citric acid)
Alka-Seltzer Morning Relief Tablets
   (aspirin, caffeine)
Alka-Seltzer PM Tablets
   (aspirin, diphenhydramine citrate)
Anacin
   (aspirin, caffeine)
Anacin-3 (Children's, Regular Strength, Maximum Strength)
   (acetaminophen)
APF Arthritis Pain Formula
   (aspirin)
Arthritis Pain Formula
   (aspirin, magnesium hydroxide, aluminum hydroxide)

aspirin

  (acetylsalicylic acid)

Aspirin-Free Arthritis Pain Formula

  (acetaminophen)

Arthropan

  (choline salicylate)

Ascriptin

  (aspirin, magnesium hydroxide, aluminum hydroxide)

Bayer: **Genuine Bayer Aspirin Tablets, Caplets, Gelcaps; Extra Strength Bayer Aspirin Caplets, Gelcaps; Aspirin Regimen Bayer Children's Chewable Tablets; Aspirin Regimen Adults Low Strength 81 mg Tablets; Aspirin Regimen Bayer Regular Strength 325 mg. Caplets; Genuine Bayer Professional Labeling (Aspirin Regimen Bayer); Extra Strength Bayer Aspirin Arthritis Caplets; Extra Strength Bayer Aspirin Caplets, Gelcaps; Bayer Plus Buffered Aspirin Gelcaps**

  (aspirin)

Bayer: **Extra Strength Bayer PM Caplets**

  (aspirin, diphenhydramine citrate)

Bayer: **Bayer Women's Aspirin Plus Calcium Caplets**

  (aspirin, calcium)

BC Powder; BC Arthritis Strength BC Powder

  (aspirin, salicylamide, caffeine)

Bufferin: **Bufferin Analgesic Capsules, Extra Strength Bufferin: Analgesic Capsules**

  (aspirin, calcium carbonate, magnesium oxide, magnesium carbonate)

Bufferin: **Bufferin Analgesic Tablets, Arthritis Strength Bufferin Analgesic Tablets, Extra Strength Bufferin Analgesic Tablets**

  (aspirin, aluminum glycinate, magnesium carbonate)

Cama

(aspirin, magnesium oxide, aluminum hydroxide)

Cosprin

(aspirin)

Easprin

(aspirin)

Ecotrin Enteric-Coated Aspirin Tablets (Low Strength, Regular Strength, Maximum Strength)

(aspirin)

Empirin

(aspirin)

Encaprin

(aspirin)

Excedrin: **Excedrin Extra Strength Tablets, Caplets, Geltabs; Excedrin Migraine Tablets, Caplets, Geltabs**

(acetaminophen, aspirin, caffeine)

Excedrin P.M.

(acetaminophen, diphenhydramine citrate)

Extra Strength Datril

(acetaminophen)

Gemnisyn

(aspirin, acetaminophen)

Goody's Body Pain Formula Powder

(aspirin, acetaminophen)

Goody's Extra Strength Headache Powder, Goody's Extra Strength Pain Relief Tablets

(aspirin, acetaminophen, caffeine)

Goody's PM Powder

(acetaminophen, diphenhydramine citrate)

Liquiprin

(acetaminophen)

Midol: Maximum Strength Midol Menstrual Caplets, Gelcaps
   (acetaminophen, pyrilamine maleate, caffeine)

Midol: Maximum Strength Midol PMS Caplets, Gelcaps
   (acetaminophen, pyrilamine maleate, pamabrom)

Midol: Maximum Strength Midol Teen Pain & Multi-Symptom Menstrual Relief Caplets
   (acetaminophen, pamabrom)

Momentum Backache Relief Extra Strength Caplets
   (magnesium salicylate tetrahydrate)

Motrin: Children's Motrin Oral Suspension, Chewable Tablets; Infants' Motrin Concentrated Drops; Junior Strength Motrin Caplets, Chewable Tablets; Motrin IB Tablets, Caplets, Gelcaps; Motrin Migraine Pain Caplets
   (ibuprofen)

Nuprin
   (ibuprofen)

Panadol, Children's Panadol
   (acetaminophen)

Percogesic: Percogesic Aspirin-Free Coated Tablets, Percogesic Extra Strength Aspirin-Free Coated Caplets
   (acetaminophen, diphenhydramine hydrochloride)

St. Joseph Aspirin for Children
   (aspirin)

St. Joseph Aspirin-Free for Children; Maximum Strength St. Joseph Aspirin-Free
   (acetaminophen)

Synalgos
   (aspirin, caffeine)

Tylenol: Children's Tylenol Suspension Liquid, Soft Chewable Tablets; Infants' Tylenol Concentrated Drops;

Junior Strength Tylenol Soft Chews Chewable Tablets;
Extra Strength Tylenol Adult Liquid Pain Reliever,
Gelcaps, Geltabs, Tablets; Regular Strength Tylenol
Tablets; Tylenol Arthritis Pain Extended Relief Caplets
(acetaminophen)

Tylenol: Women's Tylenol Multi-Symptom Menstrual
Relief Pain Reliever/Diuretic Caplets
(acetaminophen, pamabrom)

Vanquish Caplets
(aspirin, acetaminophen, caffeine)

Anesthetics

The anesthetics listed in this section block the sensation of pain.
They range from medications given to hospital patients for major
surgery, to ointments used for painful sunburns or rashes.

ANESTHETICS GIVEN IN THE HOSPITAL **UNSAFE**

The medications in this group are used to induce anesthesia, or as
part of anesthesia, and are administered most often for surgery.
They include various forms of central nervous system depressants.
They are **UNSAFE** with respect to the continued abstinence of recovering alcoholics/addicts. However, recoverees may justifiably
agree to the use of one or more of them—except nitrous oxide—
when an anesthesiologist recommends them as necessary, and sufficient caution is taken. The recovering person must be sure to
inform the anesthesiologist of his or her alcoholism/addiction and
of the possibility of an idiosyncratic reaction to the anesthesia.
(For example, some recovering individuals may be insufficiently
anesthetized by a normal dose, while others may be overanesthetized.)

Nitrous oxide is not recommended because, in the authors' opinion, it calls for special caution in order to safeguard the continued abstinence of recoverees, and it can readily be replaced by many safer and more modern anesthetics. Unlike nitrous oxide, which is inhaled as a gas, these newer anesthetics are administered either rectally or by injection.

Before being given an anesthetic, a recovering alcoholic/addict should take the following precautions:

1. Tell your doctor and the anesthesiologist about your alcoholism/ addiction, and ask for cooperation in your continued recovery. Ask them to limit anesthetics and any narcotic analgesics given postoperatively to minimum amounts and durations.
2. If time permits, plan your protection program (see "Pain," Chapter 4) with your doctors (including the anesthesiologist) before receiving the anesthetic.
3. If feasible, stay in the hospital after your surgery until all anesthetics have been eliminated from your system.

Brevital Sodium (injection)
   (methohexital sodium)
Diprivan Injectable Emulsion
   (propofol)
methohexital sodium rectal solution
nitrous oxide (inhalant gas)
Pentothal (injection or rectal suspension)
   (thiopental sodium)
Suprane
   (desflurane)
Surital
   (thiamylal sodium for injection)
thiopental sodium rectal solution

Valium Injection
(diazepam, 10% ethyl alcohol)
Versed Injection
(midazolam hydrochloride)

INHALANT ANESTHETICS GIVEN IN THE HOSPITAL **SAFE**

These anesthetics are administered by inhalation and are used most often for general anesthesia with complete unconsciousness during surgery. Some, such as Penthrane, may be given in relatively light dosages for an analgesic (pain-relieving) effect rather than as general anesthesia.

Inhalant anesthetics have little or no habit-forming effect and thus are **SAFE** for individuals recovering from substance abuse.

Ethrane
(enflurane)
Fluothane
(halothane)
Forane
(isoflurane)
halothane
Penthrane
(methoxyflurane)

OTHER ANESTHETICS GIVEN IN THE HOSPITAL **SAFE**

The anesthetics listed in this section are often used in the course of major surgery. These painkillers are termed *spinal, epidural, caudal,* or *saddle-block anesthetics* when given by a tap or injection into the lower spine. When administered in this way, these drugs act as regional or local anesthetics. A number of the anesthetics listed in this section are also given by injection in other parts of the body to produce anesthesia in those areas. Some of them are used by dentists for local anesthesia in the mouth and jaws.

Such regional or local anesthetics do not affect the entire system or influence consciousness, and they are **SAFE** for individuals recovering from substance abuse.

Carbocaine Hydrochloride
   (mepivacaine hydrochloride)
Carbocaine Hydrochloride 2 percent with Neo-Cobefrin 1:20,000 Injection
   (mepivacaine hydrochloride, levonordefrin)
Chirocaine
   (levobupivacaine hydrochloride)
Duranest Hydrochloride, Duranest Hydrochloride with Epinephrine
   (etidocaine hydrochloride, epinephrine bitartrate)
lidocaine hydrochloride injection
Marcaine Hydrochloride, Marcaine Hydrochloride with Epinephrine
   (bupivacaine hydrochloride, epinephrine bitartrate)
Marcaine Spinal
   (bupivacaine hydrochloride, dextrose)
Naropin Injection
   (ropivacaine hydrochloride)
Nesacaine, Nesacaine-MPF
   (chloroprocaine hydrochloride)
Novocain Hydrochloride for Spinal Anesthesia, Novocain Hydrochloride
   (procaine hydrochloride)
Polocaine Injection, Polocaine-MPF Injection
   (mepivacaine hydrochloride)

Pontocaine Hydrochloride for Spinal Anesthesia
(tetracaine hydrochloride)

Sarapin (injection) (relieves neuromuscular and neuralgic pain)
(sarraceniaceae plant distillate)

Sensorcaine Hydrochloride, Sensorcaine Hydrochloride with Epinephrine 1:200,000
(bupivacaine hydrochloride, epinephrine bitartrate)

Xylocaine Sterile Solution
(lidocaine hydrochloride)

Xylocaine Hydrochloride with Epinephrine
(lidocaine hydrochloride, epinephrine bitartrate)

Xylocaine Solution with Dextrose
(lidocaine hydrochloride, dextrose)

Xylocaine Solution with Glucose
(lidocaine hydrochloride, glucose)

ANESTHETICS USED IN OUTPATIENT TREATMENT **SAFE**

The anesthetics listed here are applied topically, to the skin or the mucous membranes, most often by doctors providing treatment or examination. They do not enter the system and influence consciousness or mood to any appreciable extent. They are consequently **SAFE** for recovering alcoholics or addicts.

Ophthalmologists also use topical anesthetics in examining or treating certain eye conditions. Although such infrequently encountered anesthetics are not listed here, they can also be considered safe for persons in recovery.

Americaine Anesthetic Lubricant
(benzocaine)

Analpram-HC Cream (Rectal Cream), Analpram-HC Lotion

(hydrocortisone acetate, pramoxine hydrochloride)

Anestacon

(lidocaine hydrochloride)

Cetacaine Topical Anesthetic

(benzocaine, tetracaine hydrochloride, butyl aminobanzoate)

Dyclone

(dyclonine hydrochloride)

EMLA Cream, Anesthetic Disk

(lidocaine, prilocaine)

Gebauer's Ethyl Chloride

(ethyl chloride)

Hurricaine Topical Anesthetic Spray, Gel, Liquid (nonprescription, but usually doctor-applied)

(benzocaine)

Lidoderm Patch

(lidocaine)

Pramosone Cream, Lotion

(hydrocortisone acetate, pramoxine hydrochloride)

ProctoFoam-HC

(hydrocortisone acetate, pramoxine hydrochloride)

NONPRESCRIPTION LOCAL ANESTHETICS FOR MINOR CONDITIONS **SAFE**

The following nonprescription anesthetics are applied locally to relieve minor conditions such as sunburn or other burns, rashes, hemorrhoids, mouth sores, or sore throats. Only if large amounts of the active anesthetic ingredients are absorbed into the system is there any excitant or depressant effect on the central nervous system. These medications are therefore **SAFE** for recovering individuals.

> ***Anbesol:*** **Baby Anbesol Gel, Junior Anbesol Gel, Maximum Strength Anbesol Gel, Maximum Strength Anbesol Liquid**
> *(benzocaine)*
> **Bactine Antiseptic/Anesthetic First Aid Spray**
> *(lidocaine hydrochloride, benzalkonium chloride)*
> **Betadine First Aid Antibiotics +Pain Reliever Ointment**
> *(polymyxin B sulfate, bacitracin zinc, pramoxine hydrochloride)*
> **BiCozene Creme**
> *(benzocaine, resorcinol)*
> **Campho-Phenique Cold Sore Gel, Liquid**
> *(phenol, camphor)*
> **Cepacol Anesthetic Lozenges**
> *(benzocaine, cetylpyridinium chloride)*
> **Cepastat Sore Throat Lozenges**
> *(phenol, menthol)*
> **Chloraseptic Children's Lozenges**
> *(benzocaine)*
> **Chloraseptic Lozenges, Liquid, Spray**
> *(phenol, sodium phenolate)*
> **Dermoplast Antibacterial Spray**
> *(benzocaine, benzethonium chloride)*
> **Dermoplast Pain-Relieving Spray**
> *(benzocaine, menthol)*
> **ELA-Max Cream, ELA-Max 5 Cream**
> *(lidocaine)*
> **Foille First Aid Liquid, Ointment, Spray**
> *(benzocaine, chloroxylenol)*

Herbal Ice
  (benzocaine, camphor, menthol)
Ivarest Medicated Cream, Lotion
  (benzocaine, calamine)
Kank-A Medicated Cream, Lotion
  (benzocaine, compound benzoin tincture, cetylpyridinium chloride)
Lubraseptic Jelly
  (phenyl phenol, amyl phenol)
Medicone Dressing Cream, Rectal Ointment, Rectal Suppositories
  (benzocaine, hydroxyquinoline sulfate)
Medi-Quik Aerosol Spray
  (lidocaine, benzalkonium chloride)
Nupercainal Cream, Ointment
  (dibucaine)
Orajel, Baby, Maximum Strength
  (benzocaine)
Orajel Mouth-Aid
  (benzocaine, benzalkonium chloride)
ProctoFoam (nonsteroid)
  (pramoxine hydrochloride)
Solarcaine
  (benzocaine, triclosan)
Swab and Gargle Solution
  (benzocaine, iodine, phenol, thymol)
Tronolane Anesthetic Cream, Suppositories
  (pramoxine hydrochloride)
Tronothane Hydrochloride Cream
  (pramoxine hydrochloride)
Unga-Eze
  (benzocaine, carbolic acid, zinc oxide)

Xylocaine 2.5 Ointment
  (lidocaine)
Zilactin-B Canker Sore Gel
  (benzocaine)
Zilactin Cold Sore Gel
  (benzyl alcohol)
Zilactin-L Cold Sore Liquid
  (lidocaine)

Antiallergy Medications: Antihistamines/ Antipruritics/Mast-Cell Stabilizers

The antiallergy medications described in this section are used to relieve allergic symptoms affecting the nasal membranes, bronchial passages, and eyelids—for example, runny nose, irritation, swelling, and congestion. They are also used to relieve itching and rashes, drugs that relieve itching are termed *antipruritics*.

Almost all the medications listed here are antihistamines or contain an antihistamine as an active ingredient. Most antihistamines can cause sleepiness, but people react to them in differing ways. Some don't get sleepy at all, and some get "zonked out" as if in a state of mild intoxication.

The authors believe that this last side effect is not a risk to the recovering alcoholic/addict, and that when medically appropriate, he or she can safely take antihistamines. However, there are newer antihistamines that do not have this side effect (Claritin, for example). The recovering alcoholic/addict would do well to request one of these when an antihistamine (or drug containing antihistamine) is to be prescribed.

ANTIALLERGY MEDICATIONS: PRESCRIPTION **SAFE**

Most of the antiallergy medications listed in this section are antihistamines. As previously explained, antihistamines are **SAFE** when used for the relief of allergy symptoms by individuals in recovery.

Some of the following medications contain cromolyn sodium, which is not an antihistamine but a type of drug known as a *mast-cell stabilizer*. Like antihistamines, mast-cell stabilizers reduce the effect of histamine, which causes allergic symptoms. Mast-cell stabilizers have little or no sedative properties and tend to be safe in this use by recovering alcoholics/addicts.

Alamast
   (pemirolast potassium ophthalmic solution)
Alermine
   (chlorpheniramine maleate)
Allegra Capsules, Tablets
   (fexofenadine hydrochloride)
Allegra-D Extended-Release Tablets
   (fexofenadine hydrochloride, pseudoephedrine hydrochloride)
Aller-Chlor
   (chlorpheniramine maleate)
Allerid-O.D.
   (chlorpheniramine maleate)
Alocril ophthalmic solution
   (nedocromil sodium)
Astelin Nasal Spray
   (azelastine hydrochloride)
Atrohist Sprinkle Capsules
   (brompheniramine maleate, phenyltoloxamine citrate, phenylephrine hydrochloride)

Balamine DM Oral Drops, Balamine DM Syrup
(carbinoxamine maleate, pseudoephedrine hydrochloride, dextromethorphan hydrobromide)

Bayidyl
(triprolidine hydrochloride)

Bena-D
(diphenhydramine hydrochloride)

Benadryl
(diphenhydramine hydrochloride)

Benahist
(diphenhydramine hydrochloride)

Bendylate
(diphenhydramine hydrochloride)

Bromamine
(brompheniramine maleate)

Brombay
(brompheniramine maleate)

Bromfed Capsules, Tablets; Bromfed-PD Capsules
(brompheniramine maleate, pseudoephedrine hydrochloride)

Bromphen
(brompheniramine maleate)

brompheniramine maleate tablets, elixir

Chlo-Amine
(chlorpheniramine maleate)

Chlor-100
(chlorpheniramine maleate)

Chlor-Mal
(chlorpheniramine maleate)

Chlor-Niramine
(chlorpheniramine maleate)

chlorpheniramine maleate tablets, capsules, syrup

Chlor-Pro

(chlorpheniramine maleate)

Chlorspan

(chlorpheniramine maleate)

Chlortab

(chlorpheniramine maleate)

Clarinex Tablets

(desloratadine)

Claritin Tablets, Reditabs, Syrup

(micronized loratadine)

Claritin-D 12-Hour and 24-Hour Extended Release Tablets

(loratadine, pseudoephedrine sulfate)

cyproheptadine hydrochloride tablets, syrup

Diahist

(diphenhydramine hydrochloride)

Dihydrex

(diphenhydramine hydrochloride)

Dimentabs

(diphenhydramine hydrochloride)

Diphen

(diphenhydramine hydrochloride)

Diphenacen

(diphenhydramine hydrochloride)

Diphenadril

(diphenhydramine hydrochloride)

diphenhydramine hydrochloride capsules, elixir, syrup

Dormarex

(pyrilamine maleate)

Extendryl Tablets, Capsules, Syrup

(phenylephrine hydrochloride, chlorpheniramine maleate, methscopolamine nitrate)

Fenylhist

(diphenhydramine hydrochloride)

Fynex

(diphenhydramine hydrochloride)

Gastrocrom (mast-cell stabilizer)

(cromolyn sodium)

Hal-Chlor

(chlorpheniramine maleate)

Hispril Spansule Capsules

(diphenylpyraline hydrochloride)

Histrey

(chlorpheniramine maleate)

Hydril

(diphenhydramine hydrochloride)

Hyrexin-50

(diphenhydramine hydrochloride)

Kronofed-A Kronocaps, Junior Kronofed-A Kronocaps

(pseudoephedrine hydrochloride, chlorpheniramine maleate)

Naphcon Eye Drops

(pheniramine maleate, naphazoline hydrochloride)

Nasahist B

(brompheniramine maleate)

Nasalcrom (a mast-cell stabilizer)

(cromolyn sodium)

Nolahist

(phenindamine tartrate)

Noradryl, Nordryl

(diphenhydramine hydrochloride)

Oraminic II

(brompheniramine maleate)

Opticrom ophthalmic solution (mast-cell stabilizer)

(cromolyn sodium)

Optimine Tablets
  (azatadine maleate)
Optivar ophthalmic solution
  (azelastine hydrochloride)
Patanol ophthalmic solution
  (olopatadine hydrochloride)
PBZ Elixir
  (tripelennamine citrate)
PBZ Tablets, PBZ-SR Tablets
  (tripelennamine hydrochloride, tripelenneamine citrate)
Periactin Syrup, Tablets
  (cyproheptadine hydrochloride)
Phenergan Injection, Suppositories, Tablets
  (promethazine hydrochloride)
Phenetron
  (chlorpheniramine maleate)
Polarmine Repetabs
  (dexchlorpheniramine maleate)
Robalyn
  (diphenhydramine hydrochloride)
Ryna-12 S Suspension
  (phenylephrine tannate, pyrilamine tannate)
Rynatan Pediatric Suspension
  (phenylephrine tannate, chlorpheniramine tannate)
Rynatan Tablets
  (azatadine maleate, pseudoephedrine sulfate)
Rynatuss Tablets, Pediatric Suspension
  (carbetapentane tannate, chlorpheniramine tannate, ephedrine tannate, phenylephrine tannate)
Seldane
  (terfenadine)

Semprex-D Capsules
  (acrivastine, pseudoephedrine hydrochloride)

Tacaryl Tablets, Chewable Tablets, Syrup
  (methdilazine hydrochloride)

Tavist, Tavist-1 Tablets
  (clemastine fumarate)

Tavist-D
  (clemastine fumarate, phenylpropanolamine hydrochloride)

TD Alermine
  (chlorpheniramine maleate)

Teldrin Timed-Release Allergy Capsules
  (chlorpheniramine maleate, benzyl alcohol)

Temaril Tablets, Syrup, Spansule Capsules
  (trimeprazine tartrate) (anti-itch)

tripelennamine hydrochloride tablets

triprolidine hydrochloride syrup

Trymegen
  (chlorpheniramine maleate)

Tussi-12 Tablets, Tussi-12 S Suspension
  (carbetapentane tannate, chlorpheniramine tannate)

Tusstat
  (diphenhydramine hydrochloride)

Valdrene
  (diphenhydramine hydrochloride)

Veltane
  (brompheniramine maleate)

Vistaril Capsules, Oral Suspension
  (hydroxyzine pamoate)

Wehdryl
  (diphenhydramine hydrochloride)

Zyrtec Tablets, Syrup
  (cetirizine hydrochloride)

Zyrtec-D 12-Hour Extended-Release Tablets

(cetirizine hydrochloride, pseudoephedrine hydrochloride)

ANTIALLERGY MEDICATIONS:
NONPRESCRIPTION **SAFE**

Most of the nonprescription antiallergy medications listed here contain an antihistamine as an ingredient. For relieving allergic reactions, antihistamines are **SAFE** for recovering alcoholics/addicts. Among other ingredients in these drugs are decongestants, astringents, or mild anti-irritants, all of which are safe for recovering individuals.

Take Care Not to Overuse Decongestant Nasal Sprays. An addictive-like overuse of decongestant nasal sprays can develop through carelessness. When such a spray is first used, nasal passages shrink and give relief from congestion. But the tissues then may swell more than before, leading to a second use, followed by relief and then more swelling, followed by a third use in less time than before, and so on. This is termed *rebound effect.* Such overuse can be avoided by using a decongestant nasal spray no more often and for no longer a time span than specified in the directions.

Actidil Tablets, Syrup

(triprolidine hydrochloride)

Actifed Cold and Allergy Tablets

(pseudoephedrine hydrochloride, triprolidine)

Ayr Saline Nasal Drops, Mist

(sodium chloride, water)

BC Allergy Sinus Cold Powder

(aspirin, pseudoephedrine hydrochloride, chlorpheniramine maleate)

Benadryl Allergy and Sinus Tablets, Children's Benadryl Allergy and Sinus Liquid

(diphenhydramine hydrochloride, pseudoephedrine hydrochloride)

Benadryl Allergy and Sinus Headache Caplets, Gelcaps; Benadryl Maximum Strength Severe Allergy and Sinus Headache Caplets, Gelcaps; Benadryl Allergy and Cold Caplets

(acetaminophen, diphenhydramine hydrochloride, pseudoephedrine hydrochloride)

Benadryl Allergy Ultratab Tablets; Children's Benadryl Dye-Free Allergy Liqui-Gels Softgels, Liquid Medication; Children's Benadryl Allergy Chewables, Liquid; Benadryl Allergy Kapseal Chewables

(diphenhydramine hydrochloride)

Benadryl Allergy and Sinus Fastmelt Tablets, Children's Benadryl Allergy and Cold Fastmelt Tablets

(diphenhydramine citrate, pseudoephedrine)

Bromfed Syrup

(brompheniramine maleate, pseudoephedrine hydrochloride)

Chlor-Trimeton 4-, 8-, and 12-Hour Allergy Tablets

(chlorpheniramine maleate)

Chlor-Trimeton 4- and 12-Hour Allergy/Decongestant Tablets

(chlorpheniramine maleate, pseudoephedrine sulfate)

Comtrex Sinus and Nasal Decongestant Caplets

(acetaminophen, chlorpheniramine maleate, pseudoephedrine hydrochloride)

Dimetapp Tablets, Elixir, Extentabs

(brompheniramine maleate, phenylpropanolamine hydrochloride)

Drixoral Cold and Allergy 12-Hour Sustained-Action Tablets

(dexbrompheniramine maleate, pseudoephedrine sulfate)

Fedrazil Tablets

(pseudoephedrine hydrochloride, chlorcyclizine hydrochloride)

Pediacare Cold and Allergy Liquid

(pseudoephedrine hydrochloride, chlorpheniramine maleate)

Robitussin Allergy and Cough

(brompheniramine maleate, dextromethorphan hydrobromide, pseudoephedrine hydrochloride)

Singlet Caplets

(pseudoephedrine hydrochloride, chlorpheniramine maleate, acetaminophen)

Sinutab Sinus Allergy Medication, Maximum Strength Formula, Caplets

(acetaminophen, chlorpheniramine maleate, pseudoephedrine hydrochloride)

Sudafed Sinus and Allergy Tablets

(chlorpheniramine maleate, pseudoephedrine hydrochloride)

Sudafed Sinus Nighttime

(pseudoephedrine hydrochloride, triprolidine hydrochloride)

Sudafed Sinus Nighttime Plus Pain Relief

(acetaminophen, diphenhydramine hydrochloride, pseudoephedrine hydrochloride)

Tavist 12-Hour Allergy Tablets

(clemastine fumarate)

Tavist Allergy, Sinus, Headache Caplets

(acetaminophen, clemastine fumarate, pseudoephedrine hydrochloride)

Triaminic Cold and Allergy Liquid, Softchews; Triaminic Allergy Runny Nose and Congestion Softchews

(chlorpheniramine maleate, pseudoephedrine hydrochloride)

Triaminic Allergy Congestion Softchews
 (pseudoephedrine hydrochloride)

Triaminic Allergy/Sinus/Headache Caplets
 (acetaminophen, pseudoephedrine hydrochloride)

Tylenol:

Children's Tylenol Allergy-D Liquid
 *(acetaminophen, diphenhydramine hydrochloride, pseudo-
ephedrine hydrochloride)*

**Tylenol Maximum Strength Allergy Sinus Caplets,
Gelcaps, Geltabs**
 *(acetaminophen, chlorpheniramine maleate, pseudoephedrine
hydrochloride)*

**Tylenol Maximum Strength Allergy Sinus Nite Time
Caplets**
 *(acetaminophen, diphenhydramine, pseudoephedrine hydro-
chloride)*

Tylenol Severe Allergy Caplets
 (acetaminophen, diphenhydramine)

Vicks Sinex Decongestant Nasal Spray
 (phenylephrine hydrochloride, cetylpyridinium chloride)

Vicks Sinex Long-Acting Decongestant Nasal Spray
 (oxymetazoline hydrochloride)

Visine AC Eye Drops
 (tetrahydrozoline hydrochloride, zinc sulfate)

Antiarthritic Agents SAFE

Relief of arthritic pain and/or inflammation in the joints is the main
purpose for which physicians prescribe antiarthritic drugs. Some are
also used to relieve muscular pain, pain from conditions like bursitis
and tendonitis, or pain resulting from gout. In addition, they are

sometimes prescribed to treat pain due to migraine headaches or menstruation.

The active ingredients in these medications are often safe analgesics (pain relievers) or nonsteroidal anti-inflammatory agents.

None of these medications has habit-forming or addictive effects, and thus they are all without reactivation risk for recovering alcoholics/addicts.

Celebrex *(celecoxib)*
Indocin *(indomethacin)*
Lodine *(etodolac)*
Bextra *(valdecoxib)*
Naprosyn *(naproxen)*
Vioxx *(rofecoxib)*

Antiasthmatics (Bronchodilators)

Antiasthmatics (bronchodilators) act by dilating the air passageways in the lung called *bronchioles*. Asthma attacks and some lung infections can cause the openings in the bronchiole tubes to constrict and to be further narrowed by increased mucus. Antiasthmatic drugs relieve this constriction and obstruction.

Antiasthmatics: Prescription and Nonprescription UNSAFE

The following antiasthmatic medications are **UNSAFE** for the continued abstinence of recovering alcoholics/addicts because they contain phenobarbital (an addictive barbiturate), alcohol, or both. They are prescription drugs unless otherwise noted.

Quadrinal (systemic drug, taken orally)

(ephedrine hydrochloride, phenobarbital, theophylline calcium salicylate, potassium iodide)

Tedral Elixir (a systemic drug, taken orally)

(15% alcohol, ephedrine hydrochloride, phenobarbital, theophylline)

Tedral Suspension, Tedral SA (systemic drugs, taken orally)

(ephedrine hydrochloride, phenobarbital, theophylline)

Primatene Mist (nonprescription inhalant)

(34% alcohol, epinephrine)

ANTIASTHMATICS: PRESCRIPTION AND NONPRESCRIPTION
SAFE

Antiasthmatics that do not contain barbiturates or alcohol are **SAFE** for recovering alcoholics/addicts. Before taking any antiasthmatic drug, check the ingredients to make sure it contains no possibly addictive chemicals.

INHALANT ANTIASTHMATICS

Brethaire Inhaler

(terbutaline sulfate)

Maxair Inhaler

(pirbuterol acetate)

Proventil Inhaler

(albuterol)

Ventolin Inhaler

(albuterol)

SYSTEMIC ANTIASTHMATICS

Choledyl SA Tablets

(oxtriphylline)

Lufyllin Tablets
  (dyphylline)
Slo-bid Gyrocaps
  (anhydrous theophylline)
Theo-Dur
  (anhydrous theophylline)

Antibiotics

Antibiotics are not mood-altering and are thus **SAFE** for the recovering alcoholic/addict. Antibiotics interfere with the growth of bacteria and are used to treat bacterial infections. In almost all cases, they are available only by prescription.

Macrolides are broad-spectrum antibiotics generally prescribed for respiratory-tract infections, skin and soft-tissue infections, venereal disease, and conjunctivitis, as well as urethral, endocervical, and rectal infections. Among macrolides in wide use are Erythromycin, E-Mycin, Eryc, Erythrocin Stearate, PCE, and Zithromax.

Penicillins are antibiotics that are also effective against certain respiratory tract infections, gastrointestinal and genitourinary tract infections, skin infections, and sexually transmittted diseases (STDs). They are used as well against some forms of staphylococcal and streptococcal infections. Penicillins widely used include Amcill (ampicillin), Amoxil (amoxicillin), Pentids (pencillin G potassium), and Prostaphlin (oxacillin sodium).

Tetracyclines are broad-spectrum antibiotics used with certain respiratory infections, urinary and gynecological infections, and some venereal diseases. Widely used tetracyclines include Achromycin V (tetracycline hydrochloride), Minocin (minocycline hydrochloride), and Vibramycin (doxycycline).

Cephalosporins are broad-based antibiotics prescribed mainly to fight a variety of infectious organisms within the urinary tract, respiratory tract, skin, intestinal tract, and bones and joints. They are also used for genital infections. Cephalosporins in wide use include Duricef (cefadroxil), Keflex (cephalexin), Suprax (cefixime), and Ceclor (cefaclor).

Sulfanilamides (sulfa drugs) are antibiotics commonly used for the treatment of urinary-tract infections caused by susceptible microorganisms, certain types of meningitis, and various eye and ear infections. Commonly used sulfa drugs include Bactrim (sulfamethoxazole, trimethoprim), Gantrisin (sulfisoxazole), and Septra (sulfamethoxazole, trimethoprim).

Still other types of antibiotics include: *beta-lactam antibiotics,* including Azactam (aztreonam for injection) and Lorabid (loracarbef); *aminoglycosides,* including streptomycin; and *quinolones,* including Cipro (ciprofloxacin) and Levaquin (levofloxacin).

Anticancer Agents (Antineoplastics)

Treatment of one or more types of cancer is the major purpose for which anticancer medications are used. In general, they can be obtained only by prescription.

All anticancer medications included in the following subtypes are **SAFE** for recovering alcoholics/addicts:

alkylating agents
antimetabolites
antineoplastic antibiotics
hormones
medications that reduce or stop the growth of cancerous cells

Anticancer medications in wide use include:

Adriamycin (antineoplastic antibiotic containing *doxorubicin hydrochloride*)

Leukeran (alkylating agent containing *chlorambucil*)

Tabloid (antimetabolite containing *thioguanine*)

CISplatin (antineoplastic agent containing *cisplatin*)

Myleran (alkylating agent containing *busulfan*)

Efudex (antimetabolite containing *fluorouracil*)

Mithracin (antineoplastic antibiotic containing *plicamycin*)

Aromasin (hormone containing *exemestane*)

Other drugs that are often given to recovering alcoholics/ addicts who have cancer include pain-relievers and pain-killers. (See information on analgesics earlier in this chapter.)

For important advice on actions that safeguard recovery in the case of a recovering alcoholic/addict who has cancer, see "Chronic Illness" in Chapter 4.

Anticoagulants

Anticoagulants, which reduce the ability of blood to clot, are **SAFE** for the continued abstinence of recovering alcoholics/addicts. Heparin is such a drug; another is Coumadin (crystalline warfarin sodium). Such medications are used, for example, in the treatment of phlebitis.

Anticonvulsants

In at least some applications, anticonvulsants are used to prevent convulsions in patients who have seizure disorders (including epilepsy). Anticonvulsants may be obtained only by prescription.

ANTICONVULSANTS: PRESCRIPTION **UNSAFE**

The medications in the following group are sometimes prescribed as anticonvulsants. They are **UNSAFE** for recovering alcoholics/addicts because they contain habit-forming ingredients that might reactivate addiction.

Ativan
   (lorazepam)
Klonopin
   (clonazepam)
Nembutal Sodium Solution injection
   (pentobarbital sodium)
Tranxene T-Tab; Tranxene-SD Tablets, Half-Strength Tablets
   (clorazepate dipotassium)
Valium Tablets, Injection
   (diazepam)

ANTICONVULSANTS: PRESCRIPTION **SAFE**

Because the anticonvulsants listed next do not contain habit-forming or addictive ingredients, they are **SAFE** for recovering alcoholics/addicts. In fact, some of these medications—such as phenytoin (Dilantin)—are given to alcoholics during detoxification to prevent the convulsions that sometimes result from alcohol withdrawal. A few recovering alcoholics/addicts have a tendency to suffer seizures from time to time after withdrawal, and may need to take an anticonvulsant on a continuing basis to prevent or relieve such seizures.

Carbatrol
(carbamazepine)

Celontin Capsules
(methsuximide)

Cerebyx Injection
(fosphenytoin sodium)

Depacon Injection
(valproate sodium)

Depakene Capsules, Syrup
(valproic acid)

Depakote Tablets, Depakote Sprinkle Capsules
(divalproex sodium)

Diamox Tablets, Diamox Sequels Capsules
(acetazolamide)

Dilantin Kapseals
(phenytoin sodium)

Dilantin Infatabs, Dilantin-125 Oral Suspension
(phenytoin)

Dilantin with Phenobarbital
(phenytoin, phenobarbital) (Note: Though it is a barbiturate, phenobarbital is weak in its habit-forming potential and is safe for recovering alcoholics or addicts when used as indicated here for seizure control.)

Diphenylan
(phenytoin)

Felbatol Tablets, Oral Suspension
(felbamate)

Gabitril Tablets
(tiagabine hydrochloride)

Gemonil Tablets
(metharbital)

Keppra Tablets

(levetiracetam)

Lamictal Tablets, Chewable Dispersible Tablets

(lamotrigine)

Mesantoin

(mephenytoin)

Milontin Kapseals

(phensuximide)

Mysoline

(primidone)

Neurontin Capsules, Oral Solution, Tablets

(gabapentin)

Paradione

(paramethadione)

Peganone

(ethotoin)

Phenurone Tablets

(phenacemide)

phenytoin

Tegretol Tablets, Chewable Tablets, XR Tablets, Suspension

(carbamazepine)

Topamax Tablets, Sprinkle Capsules

(topiramate)

Tridione

(trimethadione)

Trileptal Tablets, Oral Suspension

(oxcarbazepine)

Zarontin Capsules, Syrup

(ethosuximide)

Zonegran

(zonisamide)

Antidiabetics (Hypoglycemic Agents) SAFE

Control of diabetes mellitus is the main purpose for which anti-diabetics are recommended.

None of these medications tends to be habit-forming or addictive. They are therefore **SAFE** for recovering alcoholics/addicts when used as prescribed. However, taking incorrect dosages of these medications—or neglecting to take them—can result in unconsciousness or even death. Thus it is critically important to follow competent medical direction with scrupulous care when taking antidiabetics.

Among widely used antidiabetics are many brands of insulin available as prescription or nonprescription drugs taken by injection, and noninsulin prescription medications containing active ingredients such as chlorpropamide, glyburide, glipizide, and metformin, and taken orally.

Antidyskinetics (Antiparkinsonism Agents) SAFE

Antidyskinetics relieve the constant shaking, or *dyskinetics,* of the extremities, or palsy, resulting from Parkinson's disease (or parkinsonism).

These medications are also used to relieve severe side effects caused by other medicines. These include medications for treating mental illness (such as phenothiazines) or medications given to lower high blood pressure (such as reserpine).

For a recovering alcoholic/addict, any of these medications is **SAFE** when taken for its prescribed purpose, as none is habit-forming or addictive. All are available only by prescription and should be used only as prescribed. Some examples follow.

Cogentin
  (benztropine mesylate)
Artane
  (trihexyphenidyl hydrochloride)
Benadryl (given intravenously)
  (diphenhydramine hydrochloride)

Antifungal and Antiviral Agents

Clearing up fungus infections of various types—or certain viral infections—is the main purpose of antifungal and antiviral medications. For recovering alcoholics/addicts, they are all **SAFE.** Subgroups of medications of this type follow.

ANTIFUNGAL **SAFE**

SYSTEMIC
Systemic antifungal medications are generally prescribed only for deep-seated or very serious cases of fungal infections. A number of them can have serious side effects on the system. Taken by mouth or by injection and include Grifulvin V (containing griseofulvin) and Abelcet (containing amphotericin).

TOPICAL
For less serious fungal infections, topical medications are applied locally to the area affected: to the feet or the groin for complaints like athlete's foot, jock itch, or ringworm; to the vagina for various

types of vaginal infections. Topical antifungal drugs that have possibly injurious side effects can be obtained only by prescription (for example, those containing itraconazole or terbinafine). Others with milder effects are nonprescription drugs, such as Desenex, containing miconazole nitrate, and Lotrimin AF, containing clotrimazole.

ANTIVIRAL **SAFE**

Antiviral medications are prescribed to relieve a variety of infections caused by viruses. For example, those with acyclovir as the major active ingredient are used to treat the symptoms of genital herpes. Other antivirals are prescribed for illnesses ranging from flu to shingles to AIDS.

Antigout Agents SAFE

Antigout medications are prescribed to relieve or prevent gout, a painful arthritic condition of the joints that occurs chiefly in the hands, feet, and big toe. Gout results largely from a metabolic problem that causes excessive uric acid in the blood.

Antigout agents are available only by prescription, since they can have hazardous or disabling side effects. However, none of them is habit-forming or addictive, and so they are **SAFE** for recovering alcoholics/addicts.

Widely used antigout agents include drugs containing as their major active ingredient allopurinol, colchicine, or probenecid. Antiarthritic medications are also widely used to treat the symptoms of gout.

Antihypertensive Agents (High Blood Pressure Medications) SAFE

Medications used to treat hypertension (abnormally high blood pressure) are **SAFE** for recovering alcoholics/addicts. The main types of antihypertensives and examples of each follow.

ACE INHIBITORS

ACE inhibitors cause blood vessels to dilate through action on enzymes in the blood.

Accupril
   (quinapril hydrochloride)
Vasotec
   (enalapril maleate)

BETA-BLOCKERS

Beta-blockers decrease the force of heart contractions.

Corgard
   (nadolol)
Inderal
   (propanolol hydrochloride)
Tenormin
   (atenolol)

CALCIUM CHANNEL BLOCKERS

Calcium channel blockers block constriction of blood vessels through action on heart muscle and smooth muscle.

Cardizem
  (diltiazem hydrochloride)
Isoptin SR
  (verapamil hydrochloride)
Procardia
  (nifedapine)

DIURETICS

Diuretics decrease blood volume through their effect on the kidneys.
hydrochlorothiazide
  (HCTZ)
Renese
  (polythiazide)
Zaroxolyn
  (metolazone)

COMBINATION ANTIHYPERTENSIVES

Lotrel
  (amlodipine besylate, benazepril hydrochloride)
Corzide
  (nadolol, bendroflumethiazide)
Ziac
  (bisoprolol fumarate, hydrochlorothiazide)

Antiplatelet Agents SAFE

Antiplatelet agents are **SAFE** for recovering alcoholics/addicts. These medications interfere with the platelet function in clotting. Studies have indicated that aspirin may interfere with clotting and with the obstruction of the arteries by cholesterol deposits that results in atherosclerosis. Commonly used types of aspirin are Bayer, Ecotrin, and Excedrin.

Corticosteroids SAFE, BUT USE CAUTION

Corticosteroids are a class of medications that are related to hormones made by the adrenal gland. These hormones play a complex role in the balance of many physiologic functions.

Medically, corticosteroids are used in multiple ways and for many different conditions. Asthma, poison ivy, lupus erythematosus, and certain types of arthritis, allergies, and multiple sclerosis are among conditions treated by corticosteroids. Corticosteroids are available as pills, as injections, and as creams and ointments.

People sometimes confuse these drugs with the other class of "steroids," the hormones used by bodybuilders and athletes to build muscle. They are not the same, and for our purposes, only corticosteroids need be discussed.

Cortisone is the best-known corticosteroid. Prednisone is an often-prescribed oral form. Cortisone and related steroids can have an effect on mood when taken internally, making the user feel "hyper," "spacy," extremely energetic, and sometimes uncomfortably "high." Some people report difficulty sleeping after taking these steroids, although they seem to require less sleep.

In general, corticosteroids often interact with mood but in a way that is safe concerning sobriety. Each individual's reaction to cortisone is different, though, and caution should be exercised when using these drugs.

Special caution should be taken by recovering alcoholics/addicts with a number of these medications because of their alcohol content, as follows.

CORTICOSTEROIDS **UNSAFE**

Prednisone Intensol
  (prednisone, 30% alcohol)
Prednisone Oral Solution
  (prednisone, 5% alcohol)
Prelone Syrup, 15 mg
  (prednisolone, 5% alcohol)

CORTICOSTEROIDS TAKEN ORALLY OR BY INJECTION **SAFE**

A-hydroCort Vials
  (hydrocortisone sodium succinate)
A-methaPred Vials
  (methylprednisolone sodium succinate)
Aristocort Tablets
  (triamcinolone)
Aristocort Vials
  (triamcinolone diacetate)
Aristospan Vials
  (triamcinolone hexacetonide)
Celestone Tablets, Syrup
  (betamethasone)
Celestone Vials
  (betamethasone sodium phosphate)
Celestone Soluspan
  (betamethasone sodium phosphate, betamethasone acetate)
Cortef Tablets
  (hydrocortisone)
Cortef Acetate Vials
  (hydrocortisone acetate suspension)

Cortef Oral Suspension
(hydrocortisone cypionate)

cortisone acetate tablets, vials

Cortone Acetate Tablets, Injection
(cortisone acetate)

Decadron Tablets, Elixir
(dexamethasone)

Decadron Phosphate Injection
(dexamethasone sodium phosphate)

Decadron-LA Suspension Vials
(dexamethasone acetate)

Delta-Cortef Tablets
(prednisolone)

Deltasone Tablets
(prednisone)

Depo-Medrol Injectable Suspension
(methylprednisolone acetate)

dexamethasone sodium phosphate

Entocort EC Capsules
(budesonide)

Florinef Acetate Tablets
(fludrocortisone acetate)

Haldrone Tablets
(paramethasone acetate)

Hexadrol Tablets
(dexamethasone)

Hexadrol Phosphate Injection Vials, Syringes
(dexamethasone sodium phosphate)

Hydeltrosoc
(prednisolone)

Hydrocortone Tablets
(hydrocortisone)

Hydrocortone Acetate Suspension
  (hydrocortisone acetate)
Hydrocortone Phosphate Injection
  (hydrocortisone sodium phosphate)
Kenalog-10, Kenalog-40
  (triamcinoline)
Medrol Tablets
  (methylprednisolone)
Pediapred Oral Solution
  (prednisolone sodium phosphate)
**prednisolone acetate vials, prednisolone sodium phosphate
  vials**
Prednisone Tablets
  (prednisone)
Prelone Syrup (5 mg)
  (prednisolone)
Solu-Cortef Vials
  (hydrocortisone sodium succinate)
Solu-Medrol Sterile Powder
  (methylprednisolone sodium succinate)

CORTICOSTEROIDS TAKEN BY INHALATION **SAFE**

Advair Diskus
  (fluticasone propionate, salmeterol xinafoate)
AeroBid Inhaler System
  (flunisolide)
Azmacort Inhalation Aerosol
  (triamcinolone acetonide)
Beclovent
  (beclomethasone dipropionate)

Beconase
(beclomethasone dipropionate)
Flovent Diskus, Inhalation Aerosol, Rotadisk
(fluticasone propionate)
Nasalide
(flunisolide)
Pulmicort Respules Inhalation Suspension, Pulmicort Turbuhaler Inhalation Powder
(budesonide)
Qvar Inhalation Aerosol
(beclomethasone dipropionate)
Resphihaler Decadron Phosphate
(dexamethasone sodium phosphate)
Vancenase
(beclomethasone dipropionate)
Vanceril Inhalation Aerosol, Double-Strength Inhalation Aerosol
(beclomethasone dipropionate)

CORTICOSTEROIDS GIVEN RECTALLY **SAFE**

Cortenema (retention enema)
(hydrocortisone)
Corticaine Suppositories
(hydrocortisone acetate)
Proctocort Suppositories
(hydrocortisone acetate)

Cough, Cold, and Other Upper Respiratory Medications

Relieving the symptoms of coughs, colds, flu, sore throats, and other ailments of the upper respiratory tract is the main purpose for which these medications are prescribed.

Most drugs in this group consist of combinations of active ingredients, each of which acts to relieve one type of symptom. A combination medicine is accordingly designed to relieve sets of symptoms characteristic of flus, colds, or sore throats. Types of ingredients common in these medications, and the symptoms they relieve, follow.

Ingredient	Symptoms Targeted
Antihistamine	Runniness of nose, inflammation of mucous membranes
Cough suppressant	Tickle or scratchiness in throat that provokes coughing
Decongestant	Swollen tissues in nose, throat, sinuses, and lungs that close down air passages for breathing
Expectorant	Thick mucus in throat
Analgesic/antipyretic	Headache, other aches or soreness, and possibly fever

Ingredients that call for caution by recovering alcoholics or addicts consist mainly of:

- *Cough suppressants* (antitussives) that are habit-forming narcotic chemicals.

- *Analgesics* (pain relievers) such as hydrocodone or codeine, that are narcotics and strongly habit-forming. Moreover, although analgesics such as aspirin and acetaminophen are not usually habit-forming, some individuals who are strongly addiction-prone abuse them by taking them to excess when not needed to relieve pain.
- *Alcohol* is included as a mild analgesic in liquid forms of some of these medications in proportions ranging from less than 1 percent to more than 25 percent. Recovering alcoholics/addicts should not take those medicines.

Many upper-respiratory medications contain an antihistamine, which can cause sleepiness. However, some people don't get sleepy at all, and some get "zonked out."

The authors believe that this effect is not a risk to recovering alcoholics/addicts, and that when medically appropriate, they can safely take antihistamines. However, there are relatively newer antihistamines that do not induce sleepiness (Claritin, for example). The recovering alcoholic/addict would do well to request one of these when necessary.

Among the many drugs for colds and general upper-respiratory conditions, a variety of side effects exists. Some decongestants can cause a jittery, hyper, or nervous feeling that is quite uncomfortable. Other combination drugs can cause a spacy or weird feeling, and, of course, some can cause sleepiness. For recovering alcoholics/addicts, the safest approach to these medications is to use them only when necessary, and to start with lower-than-normal doses. They should discuss these suggestions with their physicians.

In the lists that follow, each type of active ingredient in a medication is listed within parentheses immediately following the brand name. These ingredients are abbreviated as follows:

antihist.: antihistamine
cough supp.: cough suppressant
decong.: decongestant
expect.: expectorant

COUGH, COLD, OR OTHER UPPER-RESPIRATORY
MEDICATIONS: PRESCRIPTION **UNSAFE**

Each of the following upper-respiratory medications is **UNSAFE** for recovering alcoholics/addicts. Addictive or habit-forming ingredients in these drugs include alcohol; codeine and its compounds, including codeine phosphate and sulfate; hydrocodone compounds, including hydrocodone bitartrate; and hydromorphone compounds, including hydromorphone hydrochloride.

Actifed with Codeine Syrup (antihist., cough supp., decong.)

(4.3% alcohol, triprolidine hydrochloride, pseudoephedrine hydrochloride, codeine phosphate)

Ambenyl Syrup (antihist., cough supp.)

(5% alcohol, bromodiphenhydramine hydrochloride, codeine phosphate)

Calcidrine Syrup (cough supp., expect.)

(6% alcohol, codeine, calcium iodide)

Cetro-Cirose Liquid (cough supp., expect.)

(1.5% alcohol, codeine phosphate, potassium guaiacolsulfonate, fluid extract ipecac)

Citra Forte Syrup (cough supp., antihist.)

(2% alcohol, hydrocodone bitartrate, pheniramine maleate, pyrilamine maleate, ascorbic acid, potassium citrate)

codeine sulfate tablets (cough supp.)

Codiclear DH Syrup (cough supp., expect.)

(hydrocodone bitartrate, potassium guaiacolsulfonate)

Dilaudid Syrup (cough supp., expect.)

(5% alcohol, hydromorphone hydrochloride, guaifenesin)

Dimetane-DC Syrup (antihist., cough supp., decong.)

(0.95% alcohol, brompheniramine maleate, phenylpropanol-amine hydrochloride, codeine phosphate)

Donatussin DC Syrup (cough supp., decong., expect.)

(hydrocodone bitartrate, phenylephrine hydrochloride, guaifenesin)

Entex Liquid (decong., expect.)

(5% alcohol, phenylephrine hydrochloride, phenylpropanol-amine hydrochloride, guaifenesin)

Entuss Liquid (cough supp., expect.)

(alcohol, hydrocodone bitartrate, potassium guaiacolsul-fonate)

Entuss Tablets (cough supp., expect.)

(hydrocodone bitartrate, guaifenesin)

Entuss-D Liquid, Tablets (cough supp., decong., expect.)

(hydrocodone bitartrate, pseudoephedrine hydrochloride, guaifenesin)

Histalet X Syrup (antihist., decong., expect.)

(15% alcohol, pseudoephedrine hydrochloride, chlorpheni-ramine maleate, guaifenesin)

Histaspan-D Capsules (antihist., decong., anticholinergic)

(alcohol, chlorpheniramine maleate, phenylephrine hydrochlo-ride, pyrilamine maleate)

Histaspan-Plus Capsules (antihist., decong.)

(alcohol, chlorpheniramine maleate, phenylephrine hydro-chloride)

Hycodan Tablets and Syrup (cough supp., anticholinergic)

(hydrocodone bitartrate, homatropine methylbromide)

Hycomine Compound Tablets (antihist., cough supp., decong., analgesic)

(hydrocodone bitartrate, chlorpheniramine maleate, phenyl-ephrine hydrochloride, acetaminophen, caffeine)

Hycomine Syrup, Hycomine Pediatric Syrup (cough supp., decong.)

(hydrocodone bitartrate, phenylpropanolamine hydrochloride)

Hycotuss Expectorant Syrup (cough supp., expect.)

(10% alcohol, hydrocodone bitartrate, guaifenesin)

Kwelkof Liquid (cough supp., expect.)

(hydrocodone bitartrate, guaifenesin)

Lufyllin-GG Elixir (expect.)

(17% alcohol, dyphylline, guaifenesin)

Naldecon-CX Suspension (cough supp., decong., expect.)

(codeine phosphate, phenlypropanolamine hydrochloride, guaifenesin)

Norisodrine with Calcium Iodide Syrup (expect., bron-chodilator)

(6% alcohol, isoproterenol sulfate, anhydrous calcium iodide)

Novahistine DH Liquid (antihist., cough supp., decong.)

(5% alcohol, codeine phosphate, pseudoephedrine hydro-chloride)

Novahistine Expectorant (cough supp., decong., expect.)

(7.5% alcohol, codeine phosphate, pseudoephedrine hydro-chloride, guaifenesin)

Nucofed Capsules, Syrup (cough supp., decong.)

(codeine phosphate, pseudoephedrine hydrochloride)

Nucofed Expectorant (cough supp., decong., expect.)

(12.5% alcohol, codeine phosphate, pseudoephedrine hydro-chloride, guaifenesin)

Nucofed Pediatric Expectorant (cough supp., decong., expect.)

(6% alcohol, codeine phosphate, pseudophedrine hydrochloride, guaifenesin)

Organidin Elixir (expect.)

(21.75% alcohol, iodinated glycerol)

Pediacof Syrup (antihist., cough supp., decong., expect.)

(5% alcohol, codeine phosphate, phenylephrine hydrochloride, chlorpheniramine maleate, potassium iodide)

Phenergan Syrup (cough supp.)

(7% alcohol, promethazine hydrochloride, dextromethorphan hydrobromide)

Phenergan VC (antihist., cough supp., decong., expect.)

(7% alcohol, promethazine hydrochloride, phenylephrine hydrochloride)

Phenergan VC with Codeine Syrup (antihist., cough supp., decong., expect.)

(7% alcohol, promethazine hydrochloride, phenylephrine hydrochloride, codeine phosphate)

Phenergan with Codeine Syrup (antihist., cough supp., expect.)

(7% alcohol, promethazine hydrochloride, codeine phosphate)

Phenergan with Dextromethorphan Syrup (antihist., cough supp., expect.)

(7% alcohol, promethazine hydrochloride, dextromethorphan hydrobromide)

Polaramine Syrup (antihist.)

(6% alcohol, dexchlorpheniramine maleate)

Promist HD Liquid (cough supp., decong., antihist.)

(5% alcohol, hydrocodone bitartrate, pseudoephedrine hydrochloride, chlorpheniramine maleate)

P-V-Tussin Syrup (antihist., cough supp., decong., expect.)

(5% alcohol, phenylephrine hydrochloride, pyrilamine maleate, chlorpheniramine maleate, ammonium chloride)

P-V-Tussin Tablets (antihist., cough supp., expect.)

(hydrocodone bitartrate, phenindamine tartrate, guaifenesin)

Robitussin A-C Syrup (cough supp., expect.)

(3.5% alcohol, codeine phosphate, guaifenesin)

Robitussin-DAC Syrup (cough supp., decong., expect.)

(1.45% alcohol, codeine phosphate, pseudoephedrine hydrochloride, guaifenesin)

Rondec-DM Syrup, Drops (antihist., cough supp., decong.)

(less than 0.6% alcohol, carbinoxamine maleate, pseudoephedrine hydrochloride, dextromethorphan hydrobromide)

Ru-Tuss Expectorant (antihist., cough supp., decong., expect.)

(5% alcohol, codeine phosphate, phenylephrine hydrochloride, chlorpheniramine maleate, ammonium chloride)

Ru-Tuss with Hydrocodone Liquid (antihist., cough supp., decong.)

(5% alcohol, hydrocodone bitartrate, phenylephrine hydrochloride, phenylpropanolamine hydrochloride, pheniramine maleate, pyrilamine maleate)

Ryna-C Liquid (antihist., cough supp., decong.)

(codeine phosphate, pseudoephedrine hydrochloride, chlorpheniramine maleate)

Ryna-CX Liquid (cough supp., decong., expect.)

(codeine phosphate, pseudoephedrine hydrochloride, guaifenesin)

S-T Forte Sugar-Free, Syrup (cough supp., decong., antihist., expect.)

(5% alcohol, hydrocodone bitartrate, phenylephrine hydrochloride, phenylpropanolamine hydrochloride, pheniramine maleate, guaifenesin)

terpin hydrate with codeine elixir (cough supp., expect.)

(41.5% alcohol, terpin hydrate, dextromethorphan hydrobromide, codeine)

Triaminic Expectorant with Codeine (cough supp., decong., expect.)

(5% alcohol, codeine phosphate, phenylpropanolamine hydrochloride, guaifenesin)

Tussar SF (Sugar-Free) Cough Syrup (antihist., cough supp., expect.)

(12% alcohol, codeine phosphate, chlorpheniramine maleate, guaifenesin, carbetapentane citrate, sodium citrate, citric acid, methylparaben)

Tussar-2 Cough Syrup (antihist., cough supp., expect.)

(5% alcohol, codeine phosphate, chlorpheniramine maleate, guaifenesin, carbetapentane citrate, sodium citrate, citric acid, methylparaben)

Tussend Expectorant (cough supp., decong., expect.)

(12.5% alcohol, hydrocodone bitartrate, pseudoephedrine hydrochloride, guaifenesin)

Tussend Tablets, Liquid (cough supp., decong.)

(5% alcohol, hydrocodone bitartrate, pseudoephedrine hydrochloride)

Tussionex Pennkinetic Extended Release Suspension (cough supp., antihist.)

(hydrocodone polistirex, phenyltoloxamine polistirex)

Tussi-Organidin Liquid (cough supp., expect.)

(codeine phosphate, iodinated glycerol)

Tussi-Organidin NR Liquid, Tussi-Organidin-S Liquid (cough supp., expect.)

(guaifenesin, codeine phosphate)

Tussi-Organidin NR Tablets (cough supp., expect.)

(guaifenesin)

Tussi-Organidin DM Newly Reformulated Liquid (cough supp., expect.)

(guaifenesin, dextromethorphan hydrobromide)

Tuss-Ornade Liquid (cough supp., decong.)

(5% alcohol, caramiphen edisylate, phenylpropanolamine hydrochloride)

Vicodin Tuss Syrup (cough supp., expect.)

(hydrocodone bitartrate, guaifenesin)

COUGH, COLD, OR OTHER UPPER RESPIRATORY MEDICATIONS: PRESCRIPTION **SAFE**

Generally speaking, the prescription medications in this group are **SAFE** for recovering alcoholics or addicts when taken exactly as prescribed.

Many of the medications in this group contain an antihistamine as an active ingredient. As mentioned previously, most antihistamines can cause sleepiness, but people react to them in different ways.

It is the authors' view that this effect is not a risk to the recovering alcoholic/addict, and that, when medically appropriate, the recoveree can safely take antihistamines. However, there are recently developed antihistamines that do not have this side effect (Seldane, for example). The recovering alcoholic/addict would do well to request one of these when an antihistamine (or combination drug containing antihistamine) is to be prescribed.

Moreover, with the many drugs for colds and general upper respiratory conditions, there is potential for differing side effects. Some decongestants can cause a jittery, hyper, or nervous feeling that is quite uncomfortable. Other combination drugs can cause a "spacy" or weird feeling, and, of course, some can cause sleepiness. For recovering alcoholics/addicts, the safest approach to these medications is to use them only when clearly necessary, and to start with lower-than-normal doses. These suggestions should be discussed with your physician.

A common pain-reliever/fever-reducer drug in some of these medications—either aspirin or acetaminophen—is subject to abuse by some addiction-prone persons, who take such a drug unnecessarily or to excess.

Alacol DM Syrup (antihist., decong., cough supp.)
   (dextromethorphan hydrobromide, phenylephrine hydrochloride, brompheniramine maleate)
Allegra-D Extended-Release Tablets (decong.)
   (fexofenadine hydrochloride, pseudoephedrine hydrochloride)
Balamine DM Oral Drops, Balamine DM Syrup (antihist., decong., cough supp.)
   (carbinoxamine maleate, pseudoephedrine hydrochloride, dextromethorphan hydrobromide)
Bromfed Capsules, Bromfed-PD Capsules (antihist., decong.)
   (brompheniramine maleate, pseudoephedrine hydrochloride)
Claritin-D 12-Hour Extended Release Tablets; 24-Hour Extended Release Tablets (antihist., decong.)
   (loratadine, pseudoephedrine sulfate)
Clistin-D Tablets (antihist., decong., analgesic)
   (phenylephrine hydrochloride, carbinoxamine maleate, acetaminophen)
Comhist Tablets, Comhist LA Capsules (antihist., decong.)
   (chlorpheniramine maleate, phenytoloxamine citrate, phenylephrine hydrochloride)
Deconamine Tablets; Deconamine SR Capsules, Syrup (antihist., decong.)
   (chlorpheniramine maleate, d-pseudoephedrine hydrochloride)

Delsym Syrup (cough supp.)
(dextromethorphan hydrobromide)

Entex Capsules (decong., expect.)
(phenylephrine hydrochloride, phenylpropanolamine hydrochloride, guaifenesin)

Entex LA Tablets (decong., expect.)
(phenylephrine hydrochloride, guaifenesin)

Extendryl SR/JR Extended-Release Capsules, Syrup, Chewable Tablets (antihist., decong.)
(phenylephrine hydrochloride, chlorpheniramine maleate, methscopolamine nitrate)

Fedahist Gyrocaps, Tablets, and Syrup (antihist., decong.)
(pseudoephedrine hydrochloride, chlorpheniramine maleate)

Guaifed Capsules, Guaifed-PD Capsules (decong., expect.)
(pseudoephedrine hydrochloride, guaifenesin)

Isoclor Capsules (antihist., decong.)
(chlorpheniramine maleate, pseudoephedrine hydrochloride)

Kronofed-A Kronocaps; Kronofed-A-JR Kronocaps (antihist., decong.)
(pseudoephedrine hydrochloride, chlorpheniramine maleate)

Lufyllin-GG Tablets (expect.)
(dyphylline, guaifenesin)

***Motrin*: Children's Motrin Cold Oral Suspension (decong., analgesic)**
(ibuprofen, pseudoephedrine hydrochloride)

Motrin Sinus/Headache Caplets (decong., analgesic)
(ibuprofen, pseudoephedrine hydrochloride)

Naldecon Tablets, Syrup, Pediatric Syrup, Drops (antihist., decong.)
(phenyltoloxamine citrate, chlorpheniramine maleate, phenylephrine hydrochloride, phenylpropanolamine hydrochloride)

Nolamine Tablets (antihist., decong.)

(phenindamine tartrate, chlorpheniramine maleate, phenyl-propanolamine hydrochloride)

Novafed A Capsules (antihist., decong.)

(chlorpheniramine maleate, pseudoephedrine hydrochloride)

Organidin NR Liquid (expect.)

(guaifenesin)

Organidin Tablets (expect.)

(guaifenesin)

Ornade Capsules (antihist., decong.)

(chlorpheniramine maleate, phenylpropanolamine hydrochloride)

Phenergan-D Tablets (antihist., decong.)

(promethazine hydrochloride, pseudoephedrine hydrochloride)

Pima Syrup (expect.)

(potassium iodide)

Rondec Tablets; Rondec-TR Tablets, Syrup, Drops (antihist., decong.)

(carbinoxamine maleate, pseudoephedrine hydrochloride)

Ru-Tuss 11 Capsules (antihist., decong.)

(chlorpheniramine maleate, phenylpropanolamine hydrochloride)

Ru-Tuss Tablets (antihist., decong., anticholinergic)

(chlorpheniramine maleate, phenylpropanolamine hydrochloride, phenylephrin hydrochloride, hyoscyamine sulfate, atropine sulfate, scopolamine hydrobromide)

Ryna-12 S Suspension (antihist., decong.)

(phenylephrine tannate, pyrilamine tannate)

Rynatan Pediatric Suspension (antihist., decong.)

(chlorpheniramine tannate, phenylephrine tannate)

Rynatan Tablets (antihist., decong.)

(azatadine maleate, pseudoephedrine sulfate)

Rynatuss Tablets, Pediatric Suspension (antihist., cough supp., decong.)

(chlorpheniramine tannate, phenylephrine tannate, carbetapentane tannate, ephedrine tannate)

Semprex-D Capsules (decong.)

(acrivastine, pseudoephedrine hydrochloride)

Sinubid Tablets (antihist., decong., analgesic)

(phenyltoloxamine citrate, phenylpropanolamine hydrochloride, acetaminophen)

Tavist-D Tablets (antihist., decong.)

(clemastine fumarate, phenylpropanolamine hydrochloride)

Tessalon Capsules (cough supp.)

(benzonatate)

Triaminic TR Tablets, Oral Infant Drops (antihist., decong.)

(pheniramine maleate, pyrilamine maleate, phenylpropanolamine hydrochloride)

Trinalin Repetabs (antihist., decong.)

(azatadine maleate, pseudoephedrine sulfate)

Tussi-Organidin DM Liquid (cough supp., expect.)

(dextromethorphan hydrobromide, iodinated glycerol)

Tussi-Organidin DM Newly Reformulated Tablets, Liquid (cough supp., expect.)

(guaifenesin, dextromethorphan hydrobromide)

Tussi-12 Suspension, Tablets (antihist., cough supp.)

(carbetapentane tannate, chlorpheniramine tannate)

Tylenol: Children's Tylenol Cold Suspension Liquid, Chewable Tablets; Maximum Strength Tylenol Allergy Sinus Caplets, Gelcaps, Geltabs (antihist., decong., analgesic)

(acetaminophen, chlorpheniramine maleate, pseudoephedrine hydrochloride)

Tylenol: Children's Tylenol Cold Plus Cough Suspension Liquid, Chewable Tablets; Children's Tylenol Flu Suspension Liquid; Multi-Symptom Tylenol Cold Complete Formula Caplets (antihist., decong., cough supp., analgesic)

(acetaminophen, chlorpheniramine maleate, dextromethorphan hydrobromide, pseudoephedrine hydrochloride)

Tylenol: Infants' Tylenol Cold, Decongestant and Fever Reducer Concentrated Drops; Children's Tylenol Sinus Suspension Liquid; Maximum Strength Tylenol Sinus Non-Drowsy Geltabs, Gelcaps, Caplets (decong., analgesic)

(acetaminophen, pseudoephedrine hydrochloride)

Tylenol: Infants' Tylenol Cold, Decongestant and Fever Reducer Concentrated Drops Plus Cough; Multi-Symptom Tylenol Cold Non-Drowsy Caplets, Gelcaps; Maximum Strength Tylenol Flu Non-Drowsy Gelcaps (decong., cough supp., analgesic)

(acetaminophen, dextromethorphan hydrobromide, pseudoephedrine hydrochloride)

Tylenol: Multi-Symptom Tylenol Cold Severe Congestion Non-Drowsy Caplets (decong., cough supp., expect., analgesic)

(acetaminophen, dextromethorphan hydrobromide, guaifenesin, pseudoephedrine hydrochloride)

Tylenol: Maximum Strength Tylenol Flu Night Time Liquid (antihist., decong., cough supp., analgesic)

(acetaminophen, dextromethorphan hydrobromide, doxylamine succinate, pseudoephedrine hydrochloride)

Tylenol: Maximum Strength Flu Night Time Gelcaps; Children's Allergy-D Liquid; Maximum Strength

Allergy Sinus Night Time Caplet (antihist., decong., analgesic)
(acetaminophen, diphenhydramine hydrochloride, pseudoephedrine hydrochloride)

Tylenol: **Maximum Strength Tylenol Sinus Night Time Caplet (antihist., decong., analgesic)**
(acetaminophen, doxylamine succinate, pseudoephedrine hydrochloride)

Tylenol Severe Allergy Caplets (antihist., analgesic)
(acetaminophen, diphenhydramine hydrochloride)

Tyzine Nasal Solution, Drops (decong.)
(tetrahydrozoline hydrochloride)

Zephrex Tablets, Zephrex LA Tablets (decong., expect.)
(pseudoephedrine hydrochloride, guaifenesin)

Zyrtec-D 12 Hour Extended Release Tablets (decong.)
(cetirizine hydrochloride, pseudoephedrine hydrochloride)

COUGH, COLD, OR OTHER UPPER-RESPIRATORY MEDICATIONS: NONPRESCRIPTION **UNSAFE**

Nonprescription liquid medicines commonly advised for upper-respiratory infections, particularly for coughs and sore throats, often include alcohol.

Thus the recovering alcoholic/addict should avoid these medications. With any liquid medication, always check the label, and choose one that is free of alcohol, perhaps double-checking with your pharmacist or physician to make sure it includes no alcohol (or any other habit-forming chemical).

Read labels with extreme care. For instance, Congespirin Liquid contains 10 percent alcohol and is potentially unsafe for recovering alcoholics/addicts. However, a related medicine deemed safe because it is alcohol-free has the similar name Congespirin Syrup.

Ambenyl-D Decongestant Cough Formula (cough supp., decong., expect.)

(9.5% alcohol, dextromethorphan hydrobromide, pseudoephedrine hydrochloride, guaifenesin)

Bayer Cough Syrup for Children (cough supp., decong.)

(5% alcohol, dextromethorphan hydrobromide, phenylpropanolamine hydrochloride)

Benylin Cough Syrup (antihist.)

(5% alcohol, diphenhydramine hydrochloride)

Benylin DM Syrup (cough supp.)

(5% alcohol, dextromethorphan hydrobromide)

Cheracol D Cough Formula (cough supp., expect.)

(4.75% alcohol, dextromethorphan hydrobromide, guaifenesin)

Cheracol Plus Head Cold/Cough Formula (antihist, cough supp., decong.)

(8% alcohol, chlorpheniramine maleate, dextromethorphan hydrobromide, phenylpropanolamine hydrochloride)

Chlor-Trimeton Allergy Syrup (antihist.)

(7% alcohol, chlorpheniramine maleate)

Comtrex Liquid (antihist., cough supp., decong., analgesic)

(20% alcohol, chlorpheniramine maleate, dextromethorphan hydrobromide, phenylpropanolamine hydrochloride, acetaminophen)

Congespirin for Children Aspirin-Free Liquid (decong., analgesic)

(10% alcohol, phenylpropanolamine hydrochloride, acetaminophen)

Contac Jr. Children's Cold Medicine (cough supp., decong., analgesic)

(10% alcohol, dextromethorphan hydrobromide, phenylpropanolamine hydrochloride, acetaminophen)

Contac Severe Cold Formula Night Strength (antihist., cough supp., decong., analgesic)

(25% alcohol, doxylamine succinate, dextromethorphan hydrobromide, pseudoephedrine hydrochloride, acetaminophen)

Coricidin Cough Syrup (cough supp., decong., expect.)

(less than 0.5% alcohol, dextromethorphan hydrobromide, phenylpropanolamine hydrochloride, guaifenesin)

Coryban-D Cough Syrup (cough supp., decong., expect., analgesic)

(7.5% alcohol, dextromethorphan hydrobromide, phenylephrine hydrochloride, guaifenesin, acetaminophen)

CoTylenol Liquid Cold Medication (antihist., cough supp., decong., analgesic)

(7.5% alcohol, chlorpheniramine maleate, dextromethorphan hydrobromide, pseudoephedrine hydrochloride, acetaminophen)

Cremacoat 1 Throat-Coating Cough Medicine (cough supp.)

(10% alcohol, dextromethorphan hydrobromide)

Cremacoat 2 Throat-Coating Cough Medicine (expect.)

(10% alcohol, guaifenesin)

Cremacoat 3 Throat-Coating Cough Medicine (cough supp., decong., expect.)

(10% alcohol, dextromethorphan hydrobromide, phenylpropanolamine hydrochloride, guaifenesin)

Cremacoat 4 Throat-Coating Cough Medicine (antihist., cough supp., decong.)

(10% alcohol, doxylamine succinate, dextromethorphan hydrobromide, phenylpropanolamine hydrochloride)

Daycare Liquid (cough supp., decong., analgesic)

(10% alcohol, dextromethorphan hydrobromide, phenylpropanolamine hydrochloride, acetaminophen)

Delsym Cough Formula Extended-Release Suspension (cough supp.)

(0.26% alcohol, dextromethorphan polistirex, dextromethorphan hydrobromide)

Demazin Syrup (antihist., decong.)

(7.5% alcohol, chlorpheniramine maleate, phenylephrine hydrochloride)

Dimetane Decongestant Tablets and Elixir (antihist., decong.)

(2.3% alcohol, brompheniramine maleate, phenylephrine hydrochloride)

Dimetane Elixir (antihist.)

(3% alcohol, brompheniramine maleate)

Dorcol Pediatric Cough Syrup (cough supp., decong., expect.)

(5% alcohol, dextromethorphan hydrobromide, phenylpropanolamine hydrochloride, guaifenesin)

Dristan Nasal Spray (antihist., decong.)

(0.4% alcohol, pheniramine maleate, phenylephrine hydrochloride)

Dristan Ultra Colds Formula Nighttime Liquid (antihist., cough supp., decong., analgesic)

(25% alcohol, chlorpheniramine maleate, dextromethorphan hydrobromide, pseudoephedrine hydrochloride, acetaminophen)

Hall's Menthol-Lyptus Decongestant Cough Formula (cough supp., decong.)

(22% alcohol, dextromethorphan hydrobromide, phenylpropanolamine hydrochloride)

Head & Chest Decongestant/Expectorant Cold Medicine Liquid (decong., expect.)

(5% alcohol, phenylpropanolamine hydrochloride, guaifenesin)

Naldecon-DX Pediatric Syrup (cough supp., decong., expect.)

(5% alcohol, dextromethorphan hydrobromide, phenyl-propanolamine hydrochloride, guaifenesin)

Naldecon-EX Pediatric Drops (decong., expect.)

(0.6% alcohol, phenylpropanolamine hydrochloride, guaifenesin)

Novahistine Cough and Cold Formula (antihist., cough supp., decong.)

(5% alcohol, chlorpheniramine maleate, dextromethorphan hydrobromide, pseudophedrine hydrochloride)

Novahistine Cough Formula (cough supp., expect.)

(7.5% alcohol, dextromethorphan hydrobromide, guaifenesin)

Novahistine DMX Liquid (cough supp., decong.)

(10% alcohol, dextromethorphan hydrobromide, pseudo-ephedrine hydrochloride)

Novahistine Elixir (antihist., decong.)

(5% alcohol, chlorpheniramine maleate, phenylephrine hydrochloride)

Nyquil Nighttime Colds Medicine (antihist., cough supp., decong., analgesic)

(25% alcohol, doxylamine succinate, dextromethorphan hydrobromide, pseudoephedrine hydrochloride, acetaminophen)

Pertussin Complex D Cough and Cold Formula (antihist., cough supp., decong.)

(9.5% alcohol, chlorpheniramine maleate, dextromethorphan hydrobromide, phenylpropanolamine hydrochloride)

Pertussin 8-Hour Cold Formula (cough supp.)

(9.5% alcohol, dextromethorphan hydrobromide)

Pertussin Original Wild Berry Cold Formula (cough supp., expect.)

(8.5% alcohol, dextromethorphan hydrobromide, guaifenesin)

Quelidrine Syrup (antihist., cough supp., decong., expect.)

(2% alcohol, chlorpheniramine maleate, dextromethorphan hydrobromide, phenylephrine hydrochloride, ephedrine hydrochloride)

Robitussin (expect.)

(3.5% alcohol, guaifenesin)

Robitussin Maximum Strength Cough Suppressant (cough supp.)

(alcohol, dextromethorphan hydrobromide)

Robitussin Maximum Strength Cough and Cold (decong., cough supp.)

(alcohol, dextromethorphan hydrobromide, pseudoephedrine hydrochloride)

Robitussin-CF (cough supp., decong., expect.)

(4.75% alcohol, dextromethorphan hydrobromide, phenylpropanolamine hydrochloride, guaifenesin)

Robitussin-DM (cough supp., expect.)

(1.4% alcohol, dextromethorphan hydrobromide, guaifenesin)

Robitussin Night Relief Colds Formula (antihist, cough supp., decong., analgesic)

(25% alcohol, pyrilamine maleate, dextromethorphan hydrobromide, phenylephrine hydrochloride, acetaminophen)

Robitussin-PE (decong., expect.)

(1.4% alcohol, pseudoephedrine hydrochloride, guaifenesin)

Russ-Tuss Liquid (antihist., decong.)

(5% alcohol, chlorpheniramine maleate, phenylephrine hydrochloride)

Sudafed Cough Syrup (cough supp., decong., expect.)

(2.4% alcohol, dextromethorphan hydrobromide, pseudo-ephedrine hydrochloride, guaifenesin)

terpin hydrate elixir (expect.)

(42.5% alcohol, terpin hydrate)

Triaminic Expectorant (decong., expect.)

(5% alcohol, phenylpropanolamine hydrochloride, guaifenesin)

Trind (antihist., decong.)

(5% alcohol, chlorpheniramine maleate, phenylpropanol amine hydrochloride)

Trind-DM (antihist., cough supp., decong.)

(5% alcohol, chlorpheniramine maleate, dextromethorphan hydrobromide, phenylpropanolamine hydrochloride)

Vicks Formula 44 Cough Mixture (antihist., cough supp.)

(10% alcohol, doxylamine succinate, dextromethorphan hydrobromide)

Vicks Formula 44D Decongestant Cough Mixture (cough supp., decong., expect.)

(10% alcohol, dextromethorphan hydrobromide, phenyl-propanolamine hydrochloride, guaifenesin)

Vicks 44 Cough Relief Liquid (cough supp.)

(5% alcohol, dextromethorphan hydrobromide)

Vicks 44D Cough and Head Congestion Relief Liquid (decong., cough supp.)

(alcohol, dextromethorphan hydrobromide, pseudoephedrine hydrochloride)

Vicks 44E Cough and Chest Congestion Relief Liquid (cough supp., expect.)

(5% alcohol, dextromethorphan hydrobromide, guaifenesin)

Vicks 44M Cough, Cold and Flu Relief Liquid (antihist., decong., cough supp.)

(alcohol, acetaminophen, chlorpheniramine maleate, dextromethorphan hydrobromide, pseudoephedrine hydrochloride)

Vicks NyQuil Cough Liquid (antihist., cough supp.)

(10% alcohol, dextromethorphan hydrobromide, doxylamine succinate)

Vicks NyQuil LiquiCaps, Liquid Multi-Symptom Cold/ Flu Relief (antihist., decong., cough supp.)

(10% alcohol, acetaminophen, dextromethorphan hydrobromide, doxylamine succinate, pseudoephedrine hydrochloride)

COUGH, COLD, OR OTHER UPPER RESPIRATORY MEDICATIONS: NONPRESCRIPTION **SAFE**

In general, the nonprescription medications in this group are **SAFE** for recovering alcoholics/addicts when taken as prescribed.

Many of the medications in this group contain an antihistamine as an active ingredient. Most antihistamines may cause sleepiness as a side effect. People react in differing ways with regard to this side effect. Some don't get sleepy at all, and some get "zonked out."

It is our feeling that this effect is not a risk to the recovering alcoholic/addict, and that, when medically appropriate, the recoveree can safely take antihistamines. However, there are recently developed antihistamines that do not have this side effect (Seldane, for example). The recovering alcoholic/addict would do well to request one of these when an antihistamine (or combination drug containing antihistamine) is to be prescribed.

Moreover, with the many drugs for colds and general upper respiratory conditions, there is potential for differing side effects. Some decongestants can cause a jittery, "hyper," or nervous feeling that is quite uncomfortable. Other combination drugs can cause a "spacy" or weird feeling, and, of course, some can cause sleepiness. For recovering alcoholics/addicts, the safest approach to these medications is to use them only when clearly necessary, and to start with lower-than-normal doses. These suggestions should be discussed with your physician.

A common pain-reliever/fever-reducer drug in some of these medications—which is either aspirin or acetaminophen in almost all cases—may be subject to abuse by some addiction-prone persons, who take such a drug unnecessarily or to excess.

NASAL SPRAYS CALL FOR CAUTION

Many nasal sprays act by constricting the nasal membranes. As a result of what might be called a rebound effect when the nasal spray wears off, there is often more swelling and obstruction. This leads to more and more frequent use of the nasal spray, and can in time produce addictivelike behavior. People have been known to develop into "nasal-spray addicts" as a result. Individuals recovering from alcoholism or addiction should hence be especially careful to stop use of a nasal spray if such addictivelike behavior starts to develop. However, compulsive overdependence on such nasal sprays can appear in anyone who is not careful about using the sprays according to directions.

Actifed Syrup, Actifed Cold and Allergy Tablets (antihist., decong.)
(pseudoephedrine hydrochloride, tripolidine hydrochloride)
Actifed Cold and Sinus MS Caplets (antihist., decong., analgesic)
(acetaminophen, chlorpheniramine maleate, pseudoephedrine hydrochloride)

Advil Cold and Sinus Caplets, Tablets; Advil Flu and Body Ache Caplets (decong., analgesic)

(ibuprofen, pseudoephedrine hydrochloride)

Afrin Nasal Spray, Drops (decong.)

(oxymetazoline hydrochloride)

Afrinol Repetabs Tablets (decong.)

(pseudoephedrine sulfate)

Aleve Cold and Sinus Caplets, Aleve Sinus and Headache Caplets (decong., analgesic)

(naproxen sodium, pseudoephedrine hydrochloride)

Alka-Seltzer Plus Cold Medicine (antihist., decong., analgesic)

(chlorpheniramine maleate, phenylpropanolamine hydrochloride, aspirin)

Alka-Seltzer Plus Cold and Cough Medicine Effervescent Tablets, Alka-Seltzer Plus Flu Medicine Effervescent Tablets, Alka-Seltzer Plus Cold and Sinus Effervescent Tablets, Alka-Seltzer Plus Night-Time Cold Medicine Effervescent Tablets (antihist., decong., cough supp., analgesic)

(aspirin, acetaminophen, chlorpheniramine maleate, dextromethorphan hydrobromide, doxylamine succinate, phenylephrine hydrochloride)

Alka-Seltzer Plus Cold and Cough Medicine Liqui-Gels, Alka-Seltzer Plus Flu Medicine Liqui-Gels, Alka-Seltzer Plus Cold Medicine Liqui-Gels, Alka-Seltzer Plus Cold and Sinus Medicine Liqui-Gels, Alka-Seltzer Plus Night-Time Cold Medicine Liqui-Gels (antihist., decong., cough supp., analgesic)

(acetaminophen, chlorpheniramine maleate, dextromethorphan hydrobromide, doxylamine succinate, pseudoephedrine hydrochloride)

Allerest Children's Chewable Tablets, Timed Release Capsules (antihist., decong.)

(chlorpheniramine maleate, phenylpropanolamine hydrochloride)

Allerest Headache Strength Tablets, Sinus Pain Formula Tablets (antihist., decong., analgesic)

(chlorpheniramine maleate, phenylpropanolamine hydrochloride, acetaminophen)

A.R.M. Allergy Relief Medicine Tablets (antihist., decong.)

(chlorpheniramine maleate, phenylpropanolamine hydrochloride)

Bayer Children's Cold Tablets (decong., analgesic)

(phenylpropanolamine hydrochloride, aspirin)

BC Allergy Sinus Cold Powder (decong., analgesic)

(aspirin, pseudoephedrine hydrochloride)

Benadryl Allergy and Cold Caplet, Benadryl Allergy and Sinus Headache Caplets (antihist., decong., analgesic)

(acetaminophen, diphenhydramine hydrochloride, pseudoephedrine hydrochloride)

Benadryl Allergy and Sinus Tablets, Children's Benadryl Allergy and Sinus Liquid (antihist., decong.)

(diphenhydramine hydrochloride, pseudoephedrine hydrochloride)

Benylin Adult Formula Cough Suppressant Liquid, Pediatric Cough Suppressant Liquid (cough supp.)

(dextromethorphan hydrobromide)

Benylin Expectorant (cough supp., expect.)

(dextromethorphan hydrobromide, guaifenesin)

Benzedrex Inhaler (decong.)

(propylhexadrine)

Breonesin Capsules (expect.)

(guaifenesin)

Chlor-Trimeton Allergy Tablets (antihist.)
(chlorpheniramine maleate)

Chlor-Trimeton Decongestant Tablets (antihist., decong.)
(chlorpheniramine maleate, pseudoephedrine sulfate)

Comtrex: **Maximum Strength Comtrex Acute Head Cold Caplets (antihist., decong., analgesic)**
(acetaminophen, brompheniramine maleate, pseudoephedrine hydrochloride)

Comtrex: **Maximum Strength Comtrex Flu Therapy Day Caplets (decong., analgesic)**
(acetaminophen, pseudoephedrine hydrochloride)

Comtrex: **Maximum Strength Comtrex Flu Therapy Night Caplets (antihist., decong., analgesic)**
(acetaminophen, chlorpheniramine maleate, pseudoephedrine hydrochloride)

Comtrex: **Multi-Symptom Comtrex Deep Chest Cold Softgels (decong., cough supp., expect., analgesic)**
(acetaminophen, dextromethorphan hydrobromide, guaifenesin, pseudoephedrine hydrochloride)

Comtrex: **Maximum Strength Comtrex Cold and Cough Day Caplets (decong., cough supp., analgesic)**
(acetaminophen, pseudoephedrine hydrochloride, dextromethorphan hydrobromide)

Comtrex: **Maximum Strength Comtrex Cold and Cough Night Caplets (antihist., decong., cough supp., analgesic)**
(acetaminophen, chlorpheniramine maleate, dextromethorphan hydrobromide, pseudoephedrine hydrochloride)

Comtrex: **Maximum Strength Comtrex Sinus and Nasal Decongestant Caplets (antihist., decong., analgesic)**
(acetaminophen, chlorpheniramine maleate, pseudoephedrine hydrochloride)

Congespirin Chewable Cold Tablets (decong., analgesic)
(phenylephrine hydrochloride, aspirin)

Congespirin for Children Aspirin-Free Chewable Cold Tablets (decong., analgesic)
(phenylephrine hydrochloride, acetaminophen)

Congespirin for Children Cough Syrup (cough supp.)
(dextromethorphan hydrobromide)

Contac Non-Drowsy 12-Hour Cold Caplets, Timed Release 12-Hour Cold Caplets (decong.)
(pseudoephedrine hydrochloride)

Contac Severe Cold and Flu Caplets Maximum Strength (antihist., cough supp., decong., analgesic)
(chlorpheniramine maleate, dextromethorphan hydrobromide, pseudoephedrine hydrochloride, acetaminophen)

Contac Severe Cold and Flu Caplets Non-Drowsy (decong., cough supp., analgesic)
(acetaminophen, psudoephedrine hydrochloride, dextromethorphan hydrobromide)

Coricidin ↓D↓ Cold, Flu and Sinus Tablets (antihist., decong., analgesic)
(acetaminophen, chlorpheniramine maleate, pseudoephedrine sulfate)

Coricidin HBP Cold and Flu Tablets (antihist., analgesic)
(acetaminophen, chlorpheniramine maleate)

Coricidin HBP Cough and Cold Tablets (antihist., cough supp.)
(chlorpheniramine maleate, dextromethorphan hydrobromide)

Coricidin HBP Maximum Strength Flu Tablets (antihist., cough supp.)
(acetaminophen, chlorpheniramine maleate, dextromethorphan hydrobromide)

Coryban-D Capsules (antihist., decong., caffeine)

(chlorpheniramine maleate, phenylpropanolamine hydrochloride, caffeine)

Daycare Capsules (cough supp., decong., analgesic)

(dextromethorphan hydrobromide, phenylpropanolamine hydrochloride, acetaminophen)

Demazin Repetabs Tablets, Syrup (antihist., decong.)

(chlorpheniramine maleate, phenylephrine hydrochloride)

Dimacol Capsules (cough supp., decong., expect.)

(dextromethorphan hydrobromide, pseudoephedrine hydrochloride, guaifenesin)

Dimetapp Elixir (antihist., decong.)

(brompheniramine maleate, pseudoephedrine hydrochloride)

Dimetapp DM Cold and Cough Elixir (antihist., decong., cough supp.)

(brompheniramine maleate, pseudoephedrine hydrochloride, dextromethorphan hydrobromide)

Dimetapp Nighttime Flu Syrup (antihist., decong., cough supp., analgesic)

(acetaminophen, brompheniramine maleate, dextromethorphan hydrobromide, pseudoephedrine hydrochloride)

Dimetapp Non-Drowsy Flu Syrup (decong., cough supp., analgesic)

(acetaminophen, dextromethorphan hydrobromide, pseudoephedrine hydrochloride)

Dimetapp Infant Drops Decongestant (decong.)

(pseudoephedrine hydrochloride)

Dimetapp Infant Drops Decongestant Plus Cough (decong., cough supp.)

(pseudoephedrine hydrochloride, dextromethorphan hydrobromide)

Disophrol Tablets (antihist., decong.)

(dexbrompheniramine maleate, pseudoephedrine sulfate)

Dristan Advanced Formula Tablets (antihist., decong., analgesic)

(chlorpheniramine maleate, phenylephrine hydrochloride, acetaminophen)

Dristan Long-Lasting Nasal Spray, Long-Lasting Menthol Nasal Spray (decong.)

(oxymetazoline hydrochloride)

Dristan Menthol Nasal Spray (antihist., decong.)

(pheniramine maleate, phenylephrine hydrochloride)

Dristan Ultra Colds Formula Capsules, Tablets (antihist., cough supp., decong., analgesic)

(chlorpheniramine maleate, dextromethorphan hydrobromide, pseudoephedrine hydrochloride, acetaminophen)

Drixoral Allergy Sinus Sustained-Action Tablets, Drixoral Cold and Flu Sustained-Action Tablets (antihist., decong., analgesic)

(acetaminophen, dexbrompheniramine maleate, pseudoephedrine sulfate)

Drixoral Cold and Allergy Sustained-Action Tablets (antihist., decong.)

(dexbrompheneramine maleate, pseudoephedrine sulfate)

Drixoral Nasal Decongestant Sustained-Action Non-Drowsy Tablets (decong.)

(pseudoephedrine sulfate)

Duration 12-Hour Nasal Spray (decong.)

(oxymetazoline)

Duration Mild 4-Hour Nasal Spray (decong.)

(phenylephrine hydrochloride)

Extend 12 Liquid (cough supp.)

(dextromethorphan hydrobromide)

4-Way Cold Tablets (antihist., decong., analgesic)

(chlorpheniramine maleate, phenylpropanolamine hydrochloride, aspirin)

4-Way Nasal Spray (antihist., decong.)

(pyrilamine maleate, phenylephrine hydrochloride, naphazoline hydrochloride)

4-Way Long-Acting Nasal Spray (decong.)

(oxymetazoline hydrochloride)

Halls Mentho-Lyptus Drops (Cherry, Honey Lemon, Ice Blue Peppermint, Spearmint, Strawberry) (cough supp.)

(menthol)

Halls Sugar-Free Drops (Black Cherry, Citrus Blend, Mountain Menthol); Halls Sugar Free Squares (Black Cherry, Mountain Menthol) (cough supp.)

(menthol)

Halls Plus Cough Suppressant Throat Drops (cough supp.)

(menthol, pectin)

Head & Chest Cold Medicine Tablets, Capsules (decong., expect.)

(phenylpropanolamine hydrochloride, guaifenesin)

Headway Capsules, Tablets (antihist., decong., analgesic)

(chlorpheniramine maleate, phenylpropanolamine hydrochloride, acetaminophen)

Hold Children's Lozenges (cough supp., decong.)

(dextromethorphan hydrobromide, phenylpropanolamine hydrochloride)

Hold Lozenges (cough supp.)

(dextromethorphan hydrobromide)

Neo-Synephrine solution (decong.)

(phenylephrine hydrochloride)

Neo-Synephrine 12-Hour Nasal Spray, Vapor Nasal Spray, Nose Drops, Children's Nose Drops (decong.)
(oxymetazoline hydrochloride)

Neo-Synephrine II Long-Acting Nasal Spray, Vapor Nasal Spray, Nose Drops, Children's Nose Drops (decong.)
(xylometazoline hydrochloride)

Neo-Synephrinol Day Relief Capsules (decong.)
(pseudoephedrine hydrochloride)

Nostril Nasal Decongestant (decong.)
(phenylephrine hydrochloride)

Nostrilla Long-Acting Nasal Decongestant (decong.)
(oxymetazoline hydrochloride)

NTZ Nasal Spray, Nose Drops (decong.)
(oxymetazoline hydrochloride)

Ornacol Capsules (cough supp., decong.)
(dextrometorphan hydrobromide, phenylpropanolamine hydrochloride)

Ornex Capsules (decong., analgesic)
(phenylpropanolamine hydrochloride, acetaminophen)

Otrivin Nasal Spray, Nose Drops (decong.)
(xylometazoline hydrochloride)

PediaCare Multisymptom Cold Liquid, Pediacare Night-Rest Cough-Cold Liquid (antihist., decong., cough supp.)
(pseudoephedrine hydrochloride, chlorpheniramine maleate, dextromethorphan hydrobromide)

PediaCare Cold and Allergy Liquid (antihist., decong.)
(pseudoephedrine hydrochloride, chlorpheniramine maleate)

PediaCare Infants' Drops Decongestant (decong.)
(pseudoephedrine hydrochloride)

PediaCare Infants' Drops Decongestant Cough; Pedia-Care Long-Acting Cough Plus Cold Liquid (decong., cough supp.)

(pseudoephedrine hydrochloride, dextromethorphan hydrobromide)

Primatene Tablets (decong., expect.)

(ephedrine hydrochloride, guaifenesin)

Privine Nasal Solution, Spray (decong.)

(naphazoline hydrochloride)

Pyrroxate Capsules (antihist., decong., analgesic)

(chlorpheniramine maleate, phenylpropanolamine hydrochloride, acetaminophen)

Robitussin Allergy and Cough (antihist., decong., cough supp.)

(brompheniramine maleate, dextromethorphan hydrobromide, pseudoephedrine hydrochloride)

Robitussin Cold Softgels Severe Congestion, Robitussin-PE Syrup (decong., expect.)

(guaifenesin, pseudoephedrine hydrochloride)

Robitussin Cold and Congestion Softgels, Caplets; Robitussin Cough and Cold Infant Drops; Robitussin Cough Formula (decong., cough supp., expect.)

(dextromethorphan hydrobromide, guaifenesin, pseudoephedrine hydrochloride)

Robitussin Cough Drops (Menthol Eucalyptus, Cherry, Honey-Lemon), Honey Calmers Throat Drops (cough supp.)

(menthol)

Robitussin Flu Liquid, Robitussin Honey Flu Nighttime Liquid (antihist., decong., cough supp., analgesic)

(acetaminophen, chlorpheniramine maleate, dextromethorphan hydrobromide, pseudoephedrine hydrochloride)

Robitussin Honey Cough Liquid, Robitussin Pediatric Strength Cough Suppressant (cough supp.)

(dextromethorphan hydrobromide)

Robitussin Liquid (expect.)

(guaifenesin)

Robitussin Multi-Symptom Cold and Flu Softgels, Caplets (decong., cough supp., expect., analgesic)

(acetaminophen, guaifenesin, pseudoephedrine hydrochloride, dextromethorphan hydrobromide)

Robitussin Multi-Symptom Honey Flu Liquid Formula, Non-Drowsy (decong., cough supp., analgesic)

(acetaminophen, dextromethorphan hydrobromide, pseudo ephedrine hydrochloride)

Robitussin Pediatric Cough and Cold Formula Liquid (decong., cough supp.)

(dextromethorphan hydrobromide, pseudoephedrine hydrochloride)

Robitussin Sinus and Congestion Caplets (decong., expect., analgesic)

(acetaminophen, guaifenesin, pseudoephedrine hydrochloride)

Robitussin Sugar Free Cough Liquid, Robitussin-DM, Robitussin-DM Infant Drops (cough supp., expect.)

(dextromethorphan hydrobromide, guaifenesin)

Ryna Liquid (antihist., decong.)

(chlorpheniramine maleate, pseudoephedrine hydrochloride)

Sinarest Tablets (antihist., decong., analgesic)

(chlorpheniramine maleate, phenylpropanolamine hydrochloride, acetaminophen)

Sine-Aid Sinus Headache Tablets, Extra-Strength Sine-Aid Caplets (decong., analgesic)

(pseudoephedrine hydrochloride, acetaminophen)

Sine-Off Extra-Strength Non-Aspirin Capsules (antihist., decong., analgesic)
(chlorpheniramine maleate, phenylpropanolamine hydrochloride, acetaminophen)

Sine-Off Extra-Strength No-Drowsiness Formula Capsules (decong., analgesic)
(phenylpropanolamine hydrochloride, acetaminophen)

Sine-Off Tablets—Aspirin Formula (antihist., decong., analgesic)
(chlorpheniramine maleate, phenylpropanolamine hydrochloride, aspirin)

Sinex Long-Acting Decongestant Nasal Spray (decong.)
(oxymetazoline hydrochloride)

Singlet Caplets for adults (antihist., decong., analgesic)
(pseudoephedrine hydrochloride, chlorpheniramine maleate, acetaminophen)

Sinutab Capsules, Tablets; Sinus Allergy Medication (antihist., decong., analgesic)
(chlorpheniramine maleate, pseudoephedrine hydrochloride, acetaminophen)

Sinutab 11 Maximum Strength, No-Drowsiness Formula Capsules, Tablets (decong., analgesic)
(pseudoephedrine hydrochloride, acetaminophen)

Sinutab Non-Drying Liquid Caps (decong., expect.)
(guaifenesin, pseudoephedrine hydrochloride)

Spec-T Sore Throat/Cough Suppressant Lozenges (cough supp., local anesthetic)
(dextromethorphan hydrobromide, benzocaine)

Spec-T Sore Throat/Decongestant Lozenges (decong., local anesthetic)
(phenylephrine hydrochloride, phenylpropanolamine hydrochloride, benzocaine)

St. Joseph Cold Tablets for Children (decong., analgesic)
(phenylpropanolamine hydrochloride, aspirin)

Sucrets Cold Decongestant Formula (decong.)
(phenylpropanolamine hydrochloride)

Sucrets Cough Control Formula (cough supp.)
(dextromethorphan hydrobromide)

***Sudafed:* Children's Sudafed Nasal Decongestant Liquid Medication, Chewables (decong.)**
(pseudoephedrine hydrochloride)

***Sudafed:* Children's Sudafed Cold and Cough Non-Drowsy Liquid (decong., cough supp.)**
(dextromethorphan hydrobromide, pseudoephedrine hydro chloride)

Sudafed Cold and Cough Liquid Caps (decong., cough supp., expect., analgesic)
(acetaminophen, dextromethorphan hydrobromide, guaifenesin, pseudoephedrine hydrochloride)

Sudafed Cough Syrup, Sustained-Action Capsules, Tablets; Sudafed Nasal Decongestant Caplets (decong.)
(pseudoephedrine hydrochloride)

Sudafed Non-Drying Sinus Liquid Caps (decong., expect.)
(guaifenesin, pseudoephedrine hydrochloride)

Sudafed Plus Syrup, Tablets; Sudafed Sinus and Allergy Tablets (antihist., decong.)
(chlorpheniramine maleate, pseudoephedrine hydrochloride)

Sudafed Severe Cold Caplets, Tablets (decong., cough supp., analgesic)
(acetaminophen, dextromethorphan hydrobromide, pseudoephedrine hydrochloride)

Sudafed Sinus and Cold Liquid Caps; Sudafed Sinus Headache Caplets, Tablets (decong., analgesic)
(acetaminophen, pseudoephedrine hydrochloride)

Sudafed Sinus Nighttime Tablets (antihist., decong.)

(pseudoephedrine hydrochloride, triprolidine hydrochloride)

Sudafed Sinus Nighttime Plus Pain Relief Caplets (antihist., decong., analgesic)

(acetaminophen, diphenhydramine hydrochloride, pseudoephedrine hydrochloride)

Tavist Allergy/Sinus/Headache Caplets (antihist., decong., analgesic)

(acetaminophen, clemastine fumarate, pseudoephedrine hydrochloride)

TheraFlu Maximum Strength Flu and Congestion Non-Drowsy Hot Liquid (decong., cough supp., expect., analgesic)

(acetaminophen, guaifenesin, pseudoephedrine hydrochloride, dextromethorphan hydrobromide)

TheraFlu Maximum Strength Severe Cold and Congestion Non-Drowsy Hot Liquid, Caplets (decong., cough supp., analgesic)

(acetaminophen, pseudoephedrine hydrochloride, dextromethorphan hydrobromide)

TheraFlu Regular Strength Cold and Sore Throat Night Time Medicine, Theraflu Maximum Strength Flu and Sore Throat Night Time Hot Liquid (antihist., decong., analgesic)

(acetaminophen, pseudoephedrine hydrochloride, chlorpheniramine maleate)

TheraFlu Regular Strength Cold and Cough Night Time Medicine; Theraflu Maximum Strength Flu and Cough Night Time Hot Liquid; Theraflu Maximum Strength Severe Cold and Congestion Night Time Hot Liquid,

Caplets (antihist., decong., cough supp., analgesic)

(acetaminophen, pseudoephedrine hydrochloride, chlorpheniramine maleate, dextromethorphan hydrobromide)

Teldrin Multi-Symptom Capsules (antihist., decong., analgesic)

(chlorpheniramine maleate, pseudoephedrine hydrochloride, acetaminophen)

Triaminic Allergy Congestion Liquid, Softchews (decong.)

(pseudoephedrine hydrochloride)

Triaminic Allergy, Sinus and Headache (decong., analgesic)

(acetaminophen, pseudoephedrine hydrochloride)

Triaminic Chest Congestion Liquid (decong., expect.)

(guaifenesin, pseudoephedrine hydrochloride)

Triaminic Chewable Tablets, Cold Tablets, Cold Syrup; Triaminic-12 Tablets (antihist., decong.)

(chlorpheniramine maleate, phenylpropanolamine hydrochloride)

Triaminic Cold and Allergy Liquid, Softchews; Triaminic Allergy, Runny Nose and Congestion Liquid (antihist., decong.)

(chlorpheniramine maleate, pseudoephedrine hydrochloride)

Triaminic Cold and Cough Liquid, Softchews; Triaminic Cold and Night Time Cough Liquid, Softchews (antihist., decong., cough supp.)

(chlorpheniramine maleate, dextromethorphan hydrobromide, pseudoephedrine hydrochloride)

Triaminic Cough Softchews (cough supp.)

(dextromethorphan hydrobromide)

Triaminic Cough Liquid, Triaminic Cough and Congestion Liquid (decong., cough supp.)

(dextromethorphan hydrobromide, pseudoephedrine hydrochloride)

Triaminic Cough and Sore Throat Liquid, Softchews (decong., cough supp.)

(acetaminophen, pseudoephedrine hydrochloride, dextromethorphan hydrobromide)

Triaminic-DM Cough Formula (cough supp., decong.)

(dextromethorphan hydrobromide, phenylpropanolamine hydrochloride)

Triaminic Flu, Cough and Fever (antihist., decong., cough supp., analgesic)

(acetaminophen, chlorpheniramine maleate, dextromethorphan hydrobromide, pseudoephedrine hydrochloride)

Triaminic Vapor Patch (cough supp.)

(camphor, menthol)

Triaminicin Tablets (antihist., decong., analgesic, caffeine)

(chlorpheniramine maleate, phenylpropanolamine hydrochloride, aspirin, caffeine)

Triaminicol Multi-Symptom Cold Tablets, Syrup (antihist., cough supp., decong.)

(chlorpheniramine maleate, dextromethorphan hydrobromide, phenylpropanolamine hydrochloride)

Tussagesic Suspension, Tablets (antihist., cough supp., decong., expect., analgesic)

(pheniramine maleate, pyrilamine maleate, dextromethorphan hydrobromide, phenylpropanolamine hydrochloride, terpin hydrate, acetaminophen)

Tylenol Maximum Strength Sinus Medication, Capsules, Tablets (decong., analgesic)

(pseudoephedrine hydrochloride, acetaminophen)

Ursinus Inlay-Tabs (antihist., decong., analgesic)

(pheniramine maleate, pyrilamine maleate, phenylpropanolamine hydrochloride, aspirin)

Vatronol Nose Drops (decong.)

(ephedrine sulfate)

Vicks Cough Drops, Menthol and Cherry Flavors (cough supp.)

(menthol)

Vicks Cough Silencers Cough Drops (cough supp., local anesthetic)

(dextromethorphan hydrobromide, benzocaine)

Vicks DayQuil LiquiCaps, Liquid Multi-Symptom Cold/ Flu Relief (decong., cough supp., analgesic)

(acetaminophen, dextromethorphan hydrobromide, pseudo-ephedrine hydrochloride)

Vicks Formula 44 Discs (cough supp., local anesthetic)

(dextromethorphan hydrobromide, benzocaine)

Vicks Inhaler (decong.)

(1-desoxyephedrine)

Vicks Pediatric 44E Cough and Chest Congestion Relief (cough supp., expect.)

(dextromethorphan hydrobromide, guaifenesin)

Vicks Pediatric 44M Cough and Cold Relief, Children's Vicks NyQuil Cold/Cough Relief (antihist., decong., cough supp.)

(chlorpheniramine maleate, dextromethorphan hydrobromide, pseudoephedrine hydrochloride)

Vicks VapoRub Ointment, Cream (decong., cough supp.)

(camphor, eucalyptus, menthol)

Vicks VapoSteam (cough supp.)

(camphor)

Dental Preparations (Mouthwash, etc.)

DENTAL PREPARATIONS: NONPRESCRIPTION **UNSAFE**

The nonprescription dental preparations listed here are **UN-SAFE** for recovering alcoholics/addicts because they contain alcohol. In general, alcoholics/addicts should always examine the labels on mouthwash bottles and use only those that are alcohol-free.

Anbesol Gel Antiseptic Anesthetic
(benzocaine, phenol, 70% alcohol)
Point-Two Dental Rinse
(sodium fluoride, 6% alcohol)

DENTAL PREPARATIONS: NONPRESCRIPTION **SAFE**

The nonprescription dental preparations that follow are **SAFE** for recovering alcoholics/addicts. Included here are oral anesthetics and antiseptics.

Chloraseptic Liquid
(phenol, sodium phenolate)
Hurricaine Topical Anesthetic
(benzocaine)
Listerine Alcohol-Free Mouthwash
(sodium lauryl sulfate, sodium benzoate, sodium saccharin, benzoic acid, zinc chloride)

Diagnostics SAFE

All diagnostic medications are **SAFE** for recovering alcoholics/addicts.

Certain diagnostic medications are ingested, including drugs such as Adenoscan and GlucaGen that stimulate or inhibit the adrenal cortex to test for adrenal corticosteroid production. Among other diagnostics that are swallowed or injected are sera for allergy skin tests, radiographic contrast media for special X-rays such as angiography, liothyronine to diagnose thyroid troubles, and drugs for testing renal function.

Diuretics (Water Pills) SAFE

Diuretics pose no risk to the sobriety of recovering alcoholics/addicts. They are used to decrease the amount of salt and water in the tissues, which when excessive is called *edema*. They accomplish this in part by increasing urinary output. Edema can be due to such conditions as congestive heart failure, hepatic cirrhosis, and the aftereffects of corticosteroid and estrogen therapy. Diuretics are also used by women to treat excess water retention prior to menstruation and are commonly used to treat high blood pressure. Some examples follow.

Hydrochlorothiazide (HCTZ)
Edecrin
   (ethacrynic acid)
Maxzide
   (triamterene, hydrochlorothiazide)

Gastrointestinal-System Medications

ANTACIDS, ANTIFLATULANTS, DIGESTANTS

Antacids, antiflatulents, and digestants are gastrointestinal medications used to treat conditions such as acid indigestion, heartburn, upset stomach, and gastritis.

ANTACIDS, ANTIFLATULENTS, DIGESTANTS: PRESCRIPTION **CHANCY**

One digestant medication is **chancy** for recovering alcoholics/addicts because it contains phenobarbital, a potentially habit-forming barbiturate. Other active ingredients include two sulfates that relax smooth muscle tissues in the digestive tract, and two pancreatic enzymes (for persons whose pancreas produces insufficient enzymes).

This drug can be taken by recovering alcoholics/addicts provided that they (1) use it only when medically prescribed; (2) take it precisely as prescribed; and (3) stop taking it at the end of the prescribed period. Although phenobarbital has no euphoric effect at the dosage in this medicine, in larger doses it may be habit-forming.

> **Arco-Lase Plus Tablets**
> *(phenobarbital, Trizyme, Lipase, hyoscyamine sulfate, atropine sulfate)*

ANTACIDS, ANTIFLATULENTS, DIGESTANTS: PRESCRIPTION AND NONPRESCRIPTION **SAFE**

The antacid, antidigestive gas, and digestion-promoting ingredients of these gastrointestinal drugs are **SAFE** for recovering alcoholics/

addicts. Most of these medications are over-the-counter drugs, but a few are available only by prescription. Many of them are combination drugs, containing, for example, both antacid and antiflatulent ingredients. Examples include the following:

Alka-Seltzer Original Antacid and Pain Reliever Tablets
(sodium bicarbonate, aspirin, citric acid)
Maalox Antacid/Antigas Liquid
(magnesium hydroxide, aluminum hydroxide, simethicone)
Tums
(calcium carbonate)
Creon 20 Capsules
(lipase, protease, amylase)
Arco-Lase Tablets
(trizyme, lipase)
Lactaid Caplets
(lactase)

ANTIDIARRHEAL AGENTS AND ORAL ELECTROLYTE SOLUTIONS

Antidiarrheal agents are used to treat diarrhea. Patients with diarrhea may need oral electrolyte solutions to offset excessive fluid and electrolyte loss.

ANTIDIARRHEAL AGENTS: PRESCRIPTION **UNSAFE**

Antidiarrheal agents containing controlled substances such as difenoxin, diphenoxylate, and opium are **UNSAFE** for recovering alcoholics/addicts.

Donnagel-PG
(opium, kaolin, pectin, hyoscyamine sulfate, atropine sulfate, scopolamine hydrobromide)

Lomotil
(diphenoxylate hydrochloride, atropine sulfate)

Motofen Tablets
(difenoxin hydrochloride, atropine sulfate)

paregoric
(camphorated tincture of opium)

Parepectolin
(paregoric, pectin, kaolin)

ANTIDIARRHEAL AGENTS: NONPRESCRIPTION **UNSAFE**

The following antidiarrheal medication is **UNSAFE** for recovering alcoholics/addicts.

Imodium A-D Liquid
(0.5% alcohol, loperamide hydrochloride)

ANTIDIARRHEAL AGENTS: NONPRESCRIPTION **SAFE**

In this group are nonprescription antidiarrheal drugs that are **SAFE** for recovering alcoholics/addicts. Active ingredients range from digestive enzymes to bacterial flora that aid in digestion.

Charcocaps
(activated vegetable charcoal)

Diasorb
(attapulgite)

Donnagel

(kaolin, pectin, hyoscyamine, atropine, scopolamine)

Enterodophilus

(strains of Lactobacillus acidophilus *and* Lactobacillus casei, *subsp.* rhamnosus*)*

Imodium Advanced Caplets, Chewable Tablets

(loperamide hydrochloride, simethicone)

Kaopectate

(kaolin and pectin)

Lactinex

(strains of Lactobacillus acidophilus and Lactobacillus bulgaricus*)*

Mitrolan

(calcium polycarbofil)

Pepto-Bismol Liquid, Tablets, Caplets

(bismuth subsalicylate)

Rheaban Maximum Strength Tablets

(attapulgite)

ORAL ELECTROLYTE SOLUTIONS **SAFE**

Oral electrolyte solutions pose no risk to recovering alcoholics/addicts. During the course of mild to severe diarrhea, excessive amounts of water and electrolytes may be lost. Oral electrolyte solutions are designed to replace these, and they usually contain carbohydrates and ions of various kinds—ingredients such as dextrose, and compounds of potassium and sodium. Rehydralyte and Pedialyte are commonly used oral electrolyte solutions.

ANTINAUSEANTS (ANTIEMETICS AND
ANTI–MOTION SICKNESS AGENTS)

Antinauseants—also called antiemetics and anti–motion sickness agents—are generally used for relief from nausea, vomiting, motion sickness, and morning sickness.

ANTINAUSEANTS: PRESCRIPTION **UNSAFE**

The antinauseants in this group are **UNSAFE** for recovering alcoholics/ addicts. Some consist of or contain dronabinol, a controlled substance. Also called *delta-9-THC,* dronabinol is one of the major ingredients in marijuana. Its street name is *THC* or *tea.* Other medications in this group have as an active ingredient pentobarbitol, which is also a controlled substance.

Dronabinol
Marinol Capsules
   (dronabinol)
"THC"
"Tea"
Wans
   (pyrilamine maleate, pentobarbital)

ANTINAUSEANTS: PRESCRIPTION **CHANCY**

For recovering alcoholics, antinauseants in this group are without risk of reactivating addiction if used with precaution. Some antinauseants, such as Benadryl, are antihistamines, while others are antidepressants or tranquilizers. Some of these medications have noneuphoric, mood-altering effects.

As a result, recovering individuals should observe the following precautions: (1) tell their doctor with complete honesty about their alcoholism/addiction; (2) ask their doctor whether the medication can be avoided; and (3) if the medication is necessary, discontinue taking it and discard any remaining supply of it as soon as possible.

Benadryl Parenteral (injection)
  (diphenhydramine hydrochloride)
Bucladin-S Softab
  (buclizine hydrochloride)
buclizine
chlorpromazine
Compazine
  (prochlorperazine)
cyclizine
diphenhydramine hydrochloride
Emete-Con
  (benzquinamide hydrochloride)
Marezine
  (cyclizine)
metoclopramide hydrochloride
perphenazine
Phenergan
  (promethazine hydrochloride)
promethazine hydrochloride
Reglan
  (metoclopramide hydrochloride)
Thorazine
  (chlorpromazine hydrochloride)
Tigan
  (trimethobenzamide hydrochloride)
Torecan
  (thiethylperazine maleate)
triflupromazine

Trilafon

(perphenazine)

trimethobenzamide

Vesprin

(triflupromazine)

ANTINAUSEANTS: PRESCRIPTION AND
NONPRESCRIPTION **SAFE**

The following prescription and nonprescription antinauseants are
SAFE for recovering alcoholics/addicts. However, Dramamine
and drugs containing meclizine can cause drowsiness.

Antivert Tablets

(meclizine hydrochloride)

Anzemet Injection, Tablets

(dolasetron mesylate)

Bonine Chewable Tablets

(meclizine hydrochloride)

Dramamine Less Drowsy Tablets

(meclizine hydrochloride)

**Dramamine Original Formula Tablets, Chewable Formula
Tablets**

(dimenhydrinate)

Emetrol Oral Solution

(dextrose [glucose], levulose [fructose], phosphoric acid)

Kytril Injection, Tablets

(granisetron hydrochloride)

meclizine

Pepto-Bismol Original Liquid, Tablets, Caplets

(bismuth subsalicylate)

Reglan Injection, Syrup, Tablets

(metoclopramide)

Transderm Scop Transdermal Therapeutic System (a skin patch)

(transdermal scopolamine)

Zofran Injection, Oral Solution, Tablets

(ondansetron hydrochloride)

ANTIULCER, ANTISECRETORY, AND ANTISPASMODIC AGENTS

The drugs listed here are used to treat problems associated with ulcers of the gastrointestinal tract. Active ingredients in some antiulcer drugs, such as sucralfate, coat the ulcer site and protect it from digestive acids. Antisecretory agents, such as cimetidine, inhibit the release or secretion of stomach acids, pepsin, and other substances into the stomach. Antispasmodics relieve irritable bowel syndrome and spasm associated with ulcers (belladonna alkaloids such as atropine, hyoscyamine, belladonna, and scopolamine act as smooth muscle relaxants to relieve spasms of the gastrointestinal tract).

ANTIULCER, ANTISECRETORY, AND ANTISPASMODIC AGENTS: PRESCRIPTION **UNSAFE**

The medications in this group are **UNSAFE** for recovering alcoholics/ addicts because they contain addictive barbiturates (such as butabarbital), alcohol, or other possibly addictive ingredients (for example, the antianxiety drug chlordiazepoxide or the tranquilizer meprobamate).

Butibel

(belladonna extract, butabarbital sodium)

Donnatal Elixir

(23% alcohol, phenobarbital, hyoscyamine sulfate, atropine sulfate, scopolamine hydrobromide)

Levsin Drops

(5% alcohol, hyoscyamine sulfate)

Levsin Elixir

(20% alcohol, hyoscyamine sulfate)

Librax

(chlordiazepoxide hydrochloride, clidinium bromide)

Milpath

(meprobamate, tridihexethyl chloride)

Pathibamate

(meprobamate, tridihexethyl chloride)

Tagamet Liquid

(2.8% alcohol, cimetidine hydrochloride)

Zantac Syrup

(7.5% alcohol, ranitidine hydrochloride)

ANTIULCER, ANTISECRETORY, AND ANTISPASMODIC
AGENTS: PRESCRIPTION **CHANCY**

The antiulcer drugs in this group can be taken by recovering
alcoholics/addicts provided that they observe precautions: (1) use
only when medically prescribed; (2) take precisely as prescribed;
and (3) stop taking at the end of the prescribed period. Caution is
needed because these medications contain phenobarbital, a barbiturate that may be habit-forming but that has no euphoric effects
at prescribed dosages.

Antrocol

(atropine sulfate, phenobarbital)

Barbidonna

*(phenobarbital, hyoscyamine sulfate, atropine sulfate, scopol-
amine hydrobromide)*

Belap

(phenobarbital, belladonna extract)

Belladenal, Belladenal-S

   (belladonna alkaloids, phenobarbital)

Bellergal, Bellergal-S

   (phenobarbitol, ergotamine tartrate, belladonna alkaloids)

Daricon PB

   (oxyphencyclimine hydrochloride, phenobarbital)

Donnatal Tablets, Capsules, Extentabs Tablets

   (phenobarbital, hyoscyamine sulfate, atropine sulfate, scopolamine hydrobromide)

Hybephen

   (atropine sulfate, scopolamine hydrobromide, hyoscyamine sulfate, phenobarbital)

Kinesed

   (phenobarbital, hyoscyamine sulfate, atropine sulfate, scopolamine hydrobromide)

ANTIULCER, ANTISECRETORY, AND
ANTISPASMODICS: PRESCRIPTION AND
NONPRESCRIPTION **SAFE**

For recovering alcoholics/addicts, the drugs listed in this group are **SAFE.** The antispasmodic ingredients used in these medications are belladonna alkaloids, which are nonaddictive.

A-Spas

   (dicyclomine hydrochloride)

Antispas

   (dicyclomine hydrochloride)

Antrenyl

   (oxyphenonium bromide)

Axid Pulvules

   (nizatidine)

atropine sulfate

Banthine

(methantheline bromide)

Baycyclomine

(dicyclomine hydrochloride)

belladonna tincture

Bellafoline

(levorotatory alkaloids of belladonna)

Bentyl Capsules, Tablets

(dicyclomine hydrochloride)

Byclomine

(dicyclomine hydrochloride)

Cantil

(mepenzolate bromide)

Carafate Suspension, Tablets

(sucralfate)

Combid

(prochlorperazine maleate, isopropamide iodide)

Cyclocen

(dicyclomine hydrochloride)

Darbid

(isopropamide iodide)

Daricon

(oxyphencyclimine hydrochloride)

Dibent

(dicyclomine hydrochloride)

Dicen

(dicyclomine hydrochloride)

Dilomine

(dicyclomine hydrochloride)

Di-Spaz

(dicyclomine hydrochloride)

Enarax

(oxyphencyclimine hydrochloride, hydroxyzine hydrochloride)

Festalan

(lipase, amylase, protease, atropine, methyl sulfate)

Famotidine Injection

(famotidine)

Kutrase Capsules

(amylase, protease, lipase, cellulase, phenyltoloxamine sulfate, hyoscyamine sulfate)

Levbid Extended Release Tablets

(hyoscyamine sulfate)

Levsin Tablets, Injection; Levsinex Timecaps; Levsin/SL Tablets

(hyoscyamine sulfate)

Neoquess

(dicyclomine hydrochloride)

Nospaz

(dicyclomine hydrochloride)

NuLev Orally Disintegrating Tablets

(hyoscyamine sulfate)

Or-Tyl

(dicyclomine hydrochloride)

Pamine

(methscopolamine bromide)

Pathilon

(tridihexethyl chloride)

Pepcid AC Chewable Tablets, Gelcaps, Tablets; Pepcid Injection, Injection Premixed; Pepcid Tablets; Pepcid RPD Orally Disintegrating Tablets; Pepcid for Oral Suspension

(famotidine)

Pepcid Complete

(famotidine, calcium carbonate, magnesium hydroxide)

Pro-Banthine

(propantheline bromide)

Quarzan

(clidinium bromide)

Robinul Injectable

(glycopyrrolate)

Robinul and Robinul Forte

(glycopyrrolate)

scopolamine hydrobromide

Spasmoject

(dicyclomine hydrochloride)

Tagamet HB 200 Suspension, Tablets; Tagamet Injection, Tablets

(cimetidine hydrochloride)

Tral

(hexocyclium methylsulfate)

Valpin

(anisotropine methylbromide)

Vistrax

(oxyphencyclimine hydrochloride, hydroxyzine hydrochloride)

Zantac 75, 150, and 300 Tablets; Zantac 150 EFFERdose Granules, Tablets; Zantac Injection, Injection Premixed

(ranitidine hydrochloride)

LAXATIVES AND STOOL SOFTENERS **SAFE**

Laxatives and stool softeners are generally **SAFE** for recovering alcoholics/addicts, and most are available without prescription. The active ingredients in laxatives stimulate the peristaltic activity of the intestine. ExLax in pill form (sennosides) is a commonly used laxative. Stool softeners such as Colace Capsules (docusate potassium) and Senokot-S Tablets (sennosides, docusate sodium) act as surfactants, which promote the absorption of water into the stool. With laxatives in syrup or liquid forms, it is wise to check the ingredients for possible alcohol content.

Geriatric Medications SAFE

Geriatric medications are prescription drugs used to help relieve a wide variety of medical problems characteristic of old age. They are safe for the recovering alcoholic/addict.

A few examples of widely used geriatric drugs include Arlidin (nylidrin hydrochloride), which is used to dilate blood vessels, especially in the extremities, to improve blood circulation; Pavabid (papaverine hydrochloride), also for dilating blood vessels; and Hydergine (ergoloid mesylates), for the treatment of a decline in mental capacity when the cause of such decline is unknown.

Heart Disease Medications SAFE

Medications for heart disease are prescription drugs that are **SAFE** for recovering alcoholics/addicts. They consist largely of four broad types of medications: antianginal agents, antiarrhythmics, cardiac preload and afterload reducers, and cardiac glycosides. Among examples of widely used heart disease drugs are the antianginal agents Nitrostat (nitroglycerine), Inderal (propranolol hydrochloride), Isordil (isosorbide dinitrate), and Procardia (nifedipine); the antiarrhythmics Betapace (sotalol hydrochloride) and Tonocard (tocainide hydrochloride); and the cardiac glycoside Lanoxin (digoxin).

Hemorrhoidal Medications SAFE

For recovering alcoholics/addicts, drugs to treat hemorrhoidal problems are **SAFE.** Such medications are used to relieve not only the pain and itching associated with hemorrhoids, but also the discomfort resulting from proctitis, rectal surgery, cryptitis, fissures, and incomplete fistulas. Their active ingredients usually include lubricants, anti-inflammatory agents, antipruritic (anti-itch) agents, and vasoconstrictive agents. These drugs are applied locally to the affected area. Some examples follow.

> Anusol-HC Cream
> *(hydrocortisone)*
> Cortifoam
> *(hydrocortisone acetate)*
> ela-Max 5 Anorectal Cream
> *(lidocaine).*

HIV/AIDS Medications SAFE

Medications employed to treat HIV/AIDS are prescription drugs that are **SAFE** for recovering alcoholics/addicts, in the sense that they pose no risk of reactivating addiction. Medicines used to treat complications of HIV/AIDS are similarly **SAFE.** Today's recommended treatment for infection by HIV (human immunodeficiency virus) is called HAART (Highly Active Antiretroviral Therapy). It includes combinations of three or more anti-HIV drugs taken in a prescribed daily regimen. Essentially similar treatment is used for AIDS (acquired immunodeficiency syndrome), which represents an advanced stage of HIV infection. A few examples of the numerous anti-HIV/AIDS medications are Rescriptor (delavirdine), Emtriva (emtricitabine), Reyataz (atazanavir), and Fuzeon (enfuvirtide). A few examples of the many medications used to treat complications of HIV/AIDS are Serostin (somatropin), Valcyte (valganciclovir), Intron A (interferon alfa-2b), gamma globulin, and Mepron (atovaquone).

Hormones SAFE

Hormones are natural substances produced by glands in the body. As medications they include a broad range of natural and synthetic drugs and are used to treat a variety of physical disorders. They are **SAFE** for recovering alcoholics/addicts insofar as continued abstinence is concerned. Hormonal medications, most of which are prescription drugs, include androgens, estrogens, progestins, fertility inducers, prolactin inducers, and thyroid hormones. (Corticosteroids, another major type, are discussed elsewhere in this chapter.)

Commonly prescribed androgens (used to treat such conditions in men as impotence and eunuchism) include Danocrine (danazol) and DEPO-Testosterone (testosterone cypionate). In this connection, it should be mentioned that the anti-impotence medication Viagra (sildenafil citrate) is not a hormone. Note that Viagra is also safe for recovering alcoholics/addicts.

Other widely used hormonal medications are: estrogens (used for menopausal symptoms, ovarian insufficiency, and certain cancer therapies) including Premarin (conjugated estrogens) and Estrace (estradiol); progesterins (used for abnormal uterine bleeding or lack of menstrual discharge), which include Aygestin (norethindrone acetate) and Provera (medroxyprogesterone acetate); fertility inducers Clomid (clomiphene citrate) and Pergonal for Injection (menotropins); and thyroid hormones Cytomel (liothyronine sodium) and Synthroid (levothyroxine sodium).

Muscle Relaxants

Muscle relaxants are used to treat muscle strain due to injury, muscle pains or cramps, and muscular tension due to stress. (They are prescribed for muscles attached to the skeleton, rather than the muscles of internal organs.)

MUSCLE RELAXANTS: PRESCRIPTION **UNSAFE**

Addictive ingredients in the following medications are **UNSAFE** for recovering alcoholics/addicts. Diazepam, the active ingredient in the antianxiety drugs Valium and Valrelease, is an addictive controlled substance. Another active ingredient, carisoprodol, acts by blocking intraneural activity in the spinal cord. Some cases of psychological dependence and abuse with this substance have been reported.

carisoprodol
Rela
   (carisoprodol)
Soma
   (carisoprodol)
Soma Compound
   (carisoprodol, aspirin)
Soma Compound with Codeine
   (carisoprodol, aspirin, codeine phosphate)
Soprodol
   (carisoprodol)

Valium
  (diazepam)
Valrelease
  (diazepam)

MUSCLE RELAXANTS: PRESCRIPTION **SAFE**

The following muscle relaxants are **SAFE** for recovering alcoholics/ addicts. Ingredients in these drugs act in a number of different ways. For example, dantrolene controls spasticity by relaxing the contractile response of the muscle directly at the muscle itself. Cyclobenzaprine has its site of action at the brain stem to reduce muscle spasm. Orphenadrine is thought to act by analgesic properties in the brain stem.

Anectine
  (succinylcholine chloride)
Banflex
  (orphenadrine)
Botox
  (Clostridium botulinum *type A)*
chlorzoxazone
Dantrium
  (dantrolene sodium)
Delaxin
  (methocarbamol)
Disipal
  (orphenadrine)
Flexeril
  (cyclobenzaprine hydrochloride)
Flexoject
  (orphenadrine)

Flexon
(orphenadrine)
K-Flex
(orphenadrine)
Lioresal
(baclofen)
Maolate
(chlorphenesin carbomate)
Marbaxin
(methocarbamol)
methocarbamol
Myobloc
(botulinum *toxin type B)*
Myolin
(orphenadrine)
Neocyten
(orphenadrine)
Norcuron
(vecuronium bromide)
Norflex
(orphenadrine citrate)
Norgesic
(orphenadrine citrate, aspirin, caffeine)
Norgesic Forte
(orphenadrine citrate, aspirin, caffeine)
O-Flex
(orphenadrine)
Orflagen
(orphenadrine)
orphenadrine
Orphenate
(orphenadrine)

Paraflex
   (chlorzoxazone)
Parafon Forte
   (chlorzoxazone)
Quinamm
   (quinine sulfate)
Robaxin
   (methocarbamol)
Robaxisal
   (methocarbamol, aspirin)
Skelaxin
   (metaxalone)
Urispas
   (flavoxate hydrochloride)
X-Otag
   (orphenadrine)
X-Otag S.R.
   (orphenadrine)
Zanaflex
   (tizanidine hydrochloride)
Zemuron
   (rocuronium bromide)

Parasitic Disease Medications SAFE

The following drugs are **SAFE** for recovering alcoholics/addicts. These medications are of two main types: antihelminthics and scabicides/pediculicides. Antihelminthics are used to treat infestations by various types of worms (including roundworms, pinworms, threadworms, hookworms, and whipworms). They are most often prescription drugs in tablet form. Some examples follow.

Povan
   (pyrvinium)
Pin-X Pinworm Treatment
   (pyrantel pamoate)

Scabicides/pediculites are used to treat scabies (mange), head lice, and crab lice. These parasite-killing drugs are applied topically in the form of shampoos, liquids, or creams. Some are prescription drugs. Examples follow.

Lindane Lotion
   (lindane)
Rid Lice-Killing Shampoo
   (pyrethrins, piperonyl butoxide)

Potassium Supplements SAFE

Potassium supplements are **SAFE** for recovering alcoholics/addicts. Their primary active ingredient—a potassium salt—is not addictive and poses no risk to continued abstinence. Other amino acids or vitamins may be secondary ingredients. These drugs are used to offset actual or potential potassium depletion, usually through losses in the urine or stool. Many are available only by prescription. Here are some examples.

Urocit-K
   (potassium citrate)
K-Phos
   (sodium phosphate)
K-Tab
   (potassium chloride)

Psychotherapeutic Agents SAFE

Psychotherapeutic agents, or psychiatric drugs, are usually given for emotional disorders or psychotic conditions. All are available only by prescription. The major kinds of psychotherapeutic drugs are antianxiety agents (minor tranquilizers), antidepressants and antimanic agents, antipsychotics (major tranquilizers), and central nervous system (CNS) stimulants.

Note: The designation "safe" with these medications means the following: any medication so designated does not endanger the continued abstinence of recovering alcoholics/addicts only if it is medically required. No drug is without reactivation risk when taken for relaxation, tranquilization, or sleep unless it is prescribed by a physician familiar with the dynamics of addiction. Any drug taken only for the purpose of effecting a temporary change in mood is dangerous to the continued abstinence of a recovering alcoholic/addict, whether that drug be an analgesic, an antihistamine, a sedative, or a tranquilizer.

The authors are aware of the controversy in some circles of recovering alcoholics/addicts concerning psychotherapeutic medications. At issue is whether a recovering alcoholic/addict who takes these medications is as "sober" (that is, as free of addictive substances) as recoverees who use no psychotherapeutic medications. The authors believe that a recovering alcoholic/addict who takes the psychotherapeutic medications identified here as safe is completely sober in this sense if the medications taken are prescribed by a psychiatrist thoroughly familiar with addiction.

ANTIANXIETY AGENTS (MINOR TRANQUILIZERS)

Antianxiety medications are prescribed to reduce nervous tension or anxiety that continues and that troubles the patient beyond normal and objectively justified levels. Commonly called tranquilizers, in psychiatry these drugs are sometimes termed *minor tranquilizers.*

ANTIANXIETY AGENTS: PRESCRIPTION **UNSAFE**

The following antianxiety drugs are **UNSAFE** for recovering alcoholics/ addicts. Indeed, these drugs are often abused by many cross-addicted individuals.

Antianxiety medications reduce excess activity of the brain that causes tension or fear. Their effect on the central nervous system is similar to that of alcohol or drugs of abuse.

Most of these antianxiety drugs are in the chemical family called *benzodiazepines,* of which perhaps the best known is Valium (diazepam). The benzodiazepines are the most highly addictive of the medications listed here. Meprobamate, a major active ingredient in other medications listed, has a comparatively lesser addictive quality.

Ativan
   (lorazepam)
Centrax
   (prazepam)
chlordiazepoxide
Dalmane
   (flurazepam)
diazepam
Deprol
   (meprobamate, benactyzine hydrochloride)
Equanil
   (meprobamate)
Halcion
   (triazolam)

Klonopin
(clonazepam)
Libritabs
(chlordiazepoxide hydrochloride)
Librium
(chlordiazepoxide hydrochloride)
Limbitrol DS Tablets
(chlordiazepoxide, amitriptyline)
Lipoxide
(chlordiazepoxide hydrochloride)
lorazepam
Menrium
(chlordiazepoxide, esterified estrogens)
Meprospan
(meprobamate)
Miltown
(meprobamate)
Miltown 600
(meprobamate)
Murcil
(chlordiazepoxide)
Pathibamate
(tridihexethyl chloride, meprobamate)
Paxipam
(halazepam)
PMB 200 and PMB 400
(premarin, meprobate)
Reposans
(chlordiazepoxide hydrocholoride)
Restoril
(temazepam)

Serax

(oxazepam)

Sereen

(chlordiazepoxide)

SK-Lygen

(chlordiazepoxide)

Tranxene

(clorazepate dipotassium)

Tranxene-SD

(clorazepate dipotassium)

Valium

(diazepam)

Valrelease

(diazepam)

Xanax

(alprazolam)

ANTIANXIETY AGENTS: PRESCRIPTION **CHANCY**

The following antianxiety drugs are **CHANCY** but are without re-activation risk for recovering alcoholics/addicts if they are pre-scribed and taken for a purpose other than anxiety. Such purposes include nausea, and sedation in conjunction with general anesthe-sia before and after surgery. The recovering alcoholic/addict must (1) take them only for the length of time prescribed and (2) discontinue them and discard any remaining supply by the end of the time for which they are prescribed.

Atarax

(hydroxyzine hydrochloride)

Atarax 100

(hydroxyzine hydrochloride)

Durrax Tablets
(hydroxyzine hydrochloride)
Vistaril
(hydroxyzine pamoate)

ANTIDEPRESSANTS AND ANTIMANIC AGENTS

Antidepressants are used to treat conditions in which patients not only feel hopeless, despairing, and fearful without objective cause, but may also have intense apathy, thoughts of suicide, and little or no appetite or sexual interest. Antimanic agents are used to treat bipolar illness, in which periods of intense depression alternate with periods of intense elation and hyperactivity.

ANTIDEPRESSANTS: PRESCRIPTION **UNSAFE**

The following antidepressants are **UNSAFE** for recovering alcoholics/ addicts because they contain potentially addictive ingredients.

Deprol
(meprobamate, benactyzine hydrochloride)
Limbitrol (also used as an antianxiety agent)
(chlordiazepoxide, amitriptylene hydrochloride)

ANTIDEPRESSANTS: PRESCRIPTION **SAFE, WHEN MEDICALLY REQUIRED**

Antidepressants in this group have no active ingredients known to be addictive. However, they are safe only when medically required and prescribed by a physician thoroughly informed about the dynamics of addiction.

Adapin
  (doxepin hydrochloride)
Amitril
  (amitriptyline hydrochloride)
amitriptyline
Asendin
  (amoxapine)
Aventyl
  (nortriptyline hydrochloride)
Celexa
  (citalopram hydrobromide)
Desyrel
  (trazodone hydrochloride)
Elavil
  (amitriptyline hydrochloride)
Effexor XR
  (venlafaxine hydrochloride)
Emitrip
  (amitriptyline hydrochloride)
Endep
  (amitriptyline hydrochloride)
Enovil
  (amitriptyline hydrochloride)
Etrafon
  (perphenazine, amitriptyline hydrochloride)
imipramine
Janimine
  (imipramine hydrochloride)
LexaPro
  (escitalopram oxalate)
Ludiomil
  (maprotiline hydrochloride)

Marplan

(isocarboxazid)

Nardil

(phenelzine sulfate)

Norpramin

(desipramine hydrochloride)

Pamelor

(nortriptyline hydrochloride)

Parnate

(tranylcypromine sulfate)

Paxil

(paroxetine hydrochloride)

Pertofrane

(desipramine hydrochloride)

Prozac

(fluoxetine hydrochloride)

Sinequan

(doxepin hydrochloride)

SK-Amitriptyline

(amitriptyline hydrochloride)

SK-Pramine

(imipramine hydrochloride)

Surmontil

(trimipramine maleate)

Tipramine

(imipramine hydrochloride)

Tofranil

(imipramine hydrochloride)

Tofranil-PM

(imipramine pamoate)

Triavil

(perphenazine, amitriptyline hydrochloride)

Vistaril
(hydroxyzine pamoate)
Vivactil
(protriptyline hydrochloride)
Zoloft
(sertraline hydrochloride)

ANTIMANIC AGENTS: PRESCRIPTION **SAFE**

Antimanic agents in this group are **SAFE** for recovering alcoholics/ addicts.

Cibalith-S
(lithium citrate)
Depakote
(divalproex sodium)
Eskalith
(lithium carbonate)
Eskalith-CR
(lithium carbonate)
Lithane
(lithium carbonate)
lithium carbonate
lithium citrate
Lithobid
(lithium carbonate)
Lithonate
(lithium carbonate)
Lithotabs
(lithium carbonate)

MAJOR TRANQUILIZERS (ANTIPSYCHOTICS):
PRESCRIPTION **SAFE**

Major tranquilizers are used to treat severe mental illnesses that block a patient's rational thinking, understanding of reality, and normal functioning. Such illnesses include paranoia and schizophrenia.

These medications do not contain habit-forming ingredients. In addition, they do not prove attractive to individuals abusing other drugs.

Chlorazine
(prochlorperazine)
Clorazine
(chlorpromazine)
Compazine
(prochlorperazine)
Eskalith-CR
(lithium carbonate)
Etrafon Tablets
(perphenazine, amitriptyline hydrochloride)
Haldol
(haloperidol)
Loxitane
(loxapine succinate)
Loxitane C
(loxapine hydrochloride)
Loxitane IM
(loxapine hydrochloride)
Luvox
(fluvoxamine maleate)

Mellaril
(thioridazine)

Mellaril-S
(thioridazine)

Millazine
(thioridazine)

Moban
(molindone hydrochloride)

Navane
(thiothixene)

Orap
(pimozide)

Ormazine
(chlorpromazine)

Permitil
(fluphenazine hydrochloride)

Prolixin
(fluphenazine hydrochloride)

Prolixin Decanoate
(fluphenazine decanoate)

Prolixin Enanthate
(fluphenazine enanthate)

Promapar
(chlorpromazine)

Promaz
(chlorpromazine)

Prozine
(promazine)

Quide
(piperacetazine)

Raudixin
(rauwolfia serpentina)

Serentil

(mesoridazine besylate)

Sparine

(promazine hydrochloride)

Stelazine

(trifluoperazine hydrochloride)

Suprazine

(trifluoperazine)

Taractan

(chlorprothixene)

thioridazine hydrochloride

Thorazine

(chlorpromazine hydrochloride)

Thor-Prom

(chlorpromazine)

Tindal

(acetophenazine maleate)

Triavil

(perphenazine, amitriptyline hydrochloride)

Trilafon

(perphenazine)

Vesprin

(triflupromazine hydrochloride)

Central Nervous System (CNS) Stimulants

Central nervous system (CNS) stimulants are prescribed mainly for narcolepsy—a tendency to fall asleep involuntarily when well rested—and for pathological hyperactivity in children.

CNS STIMULANTS: PRESCRIPTION **UNSAFE**

The CNS stimulants in this group are **UNSAFE** for recovering alcoholics/addicts, because they contain a chemical of the amphetamine family. Amphetamines are also prescribed for weight reduction with the warning that they have a high potential for abuse. In illegal use, they are known by such street names as "speed" and "uppers." Another common name is "diet pills."

In the authors' view, there is almost no medical situation in which CNS stimulants are appropriate for a recovering alcoholic/addict. The only possible exception might be a well-established diagnosis of narcolepsy.

Adderall Tablets
> *(dextroamphetamine sulfate, amphetamine sulfate, dextroamphetamine saccharate, amphetamine aspartate)*

Adipex-P
> *(phentermine hydrochloride)*

"bennies" (street name for amphetamines)

Bontril
> *(phendimetrazine tartrate)*

Concerta Extended-Release Tablets
> *(methylphenidate hydrochloride)*

Cylert Tablets
> *(pemoline)*

Desoxyn
> *(methamphetamine hydrochloride)*

Dexosyn Gradumet Tablets
> *(methamphetamine hydrochloride)*

Dexedrine
> *(dextroamphetamine sulfate)*

dextroamphetamine sulfate
DextroStat
(dextroamphetamine sulfate)
Focalin
(dexmethylphenidate hydrochloride)
Ionamin
(phentermine)
Meridia
(sibutramine hydrochloride monohydrate)
Metadate CD Capsules, Metadate ER Tablets
(methylphenidate hydrochloride)
methamphetamine hydrochloride
Methylin Tablets, Methylin ER Tablets
(methylphenidate hydrochloride)
Provigil
(modafinil)
Ritalin Hydrochloride Tablets
(methylphenidate hydrochloride)
Ritalin-SR Tablets
(methylphenidate hydrochloride)

Sedatives/Hypnotics

A number of medications used as tranquilizers are also sometimes prescribed as sedatives. These are grouped in the section on antianxiety agents and are not listed here. Similarly, some of the sedatives listed here are sometimes prescribed as tranquilizers.

Sedatives are used to quiet the system; hypnotics are used to produce sleep. Most of the medications listed here can be used as either sedatives or hypnotics, depending on dosage.

SEDATIVES: PRESCRIPTION **UNSAFE**

The sedatives in this group might be recommended to relieve serious insomnia and/or severe nervous apprehension or anxiety. Most of them act as central nervous system depressants, dulling the brain and bringing on drowsiness. With almost any one of these sedatives, a large dose can make one unconscious; an overdose can be fatal.

In addition, for recovering alcoholics/addicts, even light dosages of these sedatives call for special caution. Almost every one is extremely habit-forming.

The addictive active ingredients are indicated in parentheses directly under the name of the medication. For generic drugs, the addictive active ingredient is the medication identified in the generic name itself.

If you are recovering from alcohol or drug abuse, *do not take any of these sedatives if you can possibly avoid doing so*. There is one exception: phenobarbital used for seizure control (See the following section on barbiturates).

Should you need relief from insomnia or anxiety, do all you can to use other means recommended in this book instead of prescription sedatives. (See Chapter four.)

BARBITURATES: PRESCRIPTION **UNSAFE**

Barbiturates have been considered classically addictive drugs for many years. Although their effects vary, most barbiturates are markedly sedating, and some also have euphoric qualities. They therefore call for special caution by recovering alcoholics/addicts.

Because barbiturates are present in common headache and pain medications, as well as in many anesthetics, you should take special care to guard against taking them by accident. Phenobarbital, when prescribed for seizure control in alcoholics, is the one exception to this warning. The most common two-drug combination prescribed for seizure control consists of phenytoin (Dilantin) and phenobarbital. Phenobarbital has very little of the sedating qualities of other barbiturates, and none of the euphoric effects.

As a result, recovering alcoholics can usually take phenobarbital for seizure control without risking reactivation of their addiction. Some recovering alcoholics who are subject to chronic seizures or convulsions are accordingly prescribed it on a continuing basis.

Phenobarbital is also often given with phenytoin for a number of days during detoxification from alcohol. This is to prevent alcohol withdrawal seizures.

Alurate Elixir
   (aprobarbital, 20% alcohol)
amobarbital
Amytal Sodium
   (amobarbital sodium)
B-A-C Tablets
   (butalbital)
butabarbital
Buticaps, Butisol Sodium Tablets, Elixir
   (sodium butabarbital: elixir also includes 7% alcohol)
Lotusate
   (talbutal)
Luminal (Note: See exception and warning about phenobarbital under "Barbiturates.")
   (phenobarbital)
Mebaral Tablets
   (mephobarbital)
Nembutal Elixir, Ampules, Vials (for injection)
   (pentobarbital, 10% alcohol)

Nembutal Sodium Capsules, Solution, Suppositories
   (pentobarbital sodium)
pentobarbital
**phenobarbital, phenobarbital sodium (Note: See exception
   and warning about phenobarbital under "Barbiturates.")**
"reds" (street name for Seconal Capsules)
secobarbital
Seconal Sodium Capsules, Injection, Suppositories
   (secobarbital sodium)
Tuinal
   (secobarbital sodium, amobarbital sodium)
"yellows" (street name for Nembutal Capsules)

OTHER SEDATIVES: PRESCRIPTION **HIGHLY UNSAFE**

Like the barbiturate sedatives, these prescription sedatives are
HIGHLY UNSAFE for recoverees. If you are recovering from alcohol or drug abuse, *do not take any of these sedatives*. Go without
sleep instead, if necessary.

Ambien Tablets
   (zolpidem tartrate)
chloral hydrate capsules, elixir, syrup, suppositories
Dalmane
   (flurazepam hydrochloride)
Diprivan Injectable Emulsion
   (propofol)
Doriden
   (glutethimide)
glutethimide
Halcion
   (triazolam)

Largon
(propiomazine hydrochloride)
"ludes" (street name for methaqualone)
Mepergan Injection
(meperidine hydrochloride, promethazine hydrochloride)
"Mickey Finn" (street name for a cocktail of chloral
hydrate capsules dissolved in high-proof alcohol)
Noctec
(chloral hydrate)
Noludar, Noludar 300
(methyprylon)
methaqualone (Once marketed with brand names that included Quaalude, Mequin, and Parest, but it is no
longer on the market; it is illegally made and sold as a
street drug.)
Phenergan Syrup Fortis
(1.5% alcohol, promethazine hydrochloride)
Phenergan Syrup Plain
(7% alcohol, promethazine hydrochloride)
Placidyl
(ethchlorvynol)
ProSom Tablets
(estazolam)
Restoril
(temazepam)
"soapers" (street name for methaqualone)
Sonata Capsules
(zaleplon)
Valmid
(ethinamate)
Versed Syrup, Injection
(midazolam hydrochloride)

SEDATIVES: NONPRESCRIPTION **UNSAFE**

The nonprescription sleep preparations listed here include antihistamines, which have a dulling or drowsiness-inducing effect. However, they seem to have little or no habit-forming effect. (See the introduction to the "Antiallergy Medications" in this chapter.)

Nevertheless, the authors believe that taking antihistamines to change one's state of consciousness (from wakefulness to sleep) offers a risk to any recovering alcoholic/addict. Such an act risks reactivating acute addiction because it may revive old patterns of addictive behavior for the purpose of changing mood (or conscious state).

Accordingly, the authors believe that taking these antihistamine preparations as sedatives is **UNSAFE** for recovering alcoholics/addicts. However, using antihistamines for other purposes—to combat allergies or upper respiratory congestion, for instance—is deemed safe, because the purpose does not involve mood-changing, and the active ingredients are not habit-forming.

Alka-Seltzer PM Tablets
   (diphenhydramine citrate, aspirin)
Bayer: **Extra Strength Bayer PM Caplets**
   (diphenhydramine citrate, aspirin)
Excedrin PM Tablets, Caplets, Gelcaps
   (diphenhydramine citrate, acetaminophen)
Goody's PM Powder
   (diphenhydramine citrate, acetaminophen)
Nervine Night-Time Sleep Aid
   (diphenhydramine)
Nytol: **Nytol QuickCaps Caplets, Maximum Strength Nytol QuickGels Softgels**
   (diphenhydramine hydrochloride)

Simply Sleep Caplets
(diphenhydramine hydrochloride)

Sleep-Eze Tablets
(diphenhydramine hydrochloride)

Sominex Original Formula Tablets
(diphenhydramine hydrochloride)

Unisom Maximum Strength SleepGels
(diphenhydramine hydrochloride)

Unisom SleepTabs
(doxylamine succinate)

Serum Cholesterol-Lowering and Fat-Lowering Medications (Hypolipidemics) SAFE

Hypolipidemics reduce the levels of cholesterol and triglycerides in the blood. Cholesterol and triglycerides are fats that are thought to contribute to the development of atherosclerosis and related cardiovascular disease, such as heart attacks and strokes. These medications are **SAFE** for recovering alcoholics/addicts.

Lopid
(gemfibrozil)
Mevacor
(lovastatin)
Lescol
(fluvastatin sodium)

Urinary-Tract Agents

Urinary-tract medications combat infections (anti-infectives), relieve pain (analgesics), relax constriction (antispasmodics), and improve urinary retention (parasympathomimetics). They are generally prescription drugs.

URINARY-TRACT AGENTS: PRESCRIPTION **UNSAFE**

The urinary analgesic listed here is **UNSAFE** for recovering alcoholics/ addicts. It contains butabarbital, a barbiturate that is an addictive controlled substance.

Pyridium Plus
(phenazopyridine hydrochloride, hyoscyamine hydrobromide, butabarbital)

URINARY-TRACT AGENTS: PRESCRIPTION **SAFE**

Urinary-tract medications are **SAFE** for the recovering alcoholic/ addict when they contain no mood-altering ingredients. Urinary anti-infectives generally have bactericidal ingredients such as sulfonamides for the treatment of uncomplicated urinary infections. Two examples follow.

Bactrim
(trimethoprim, sulfamethoxazole)
Macrodantin
(nitrofurantoin macrocrystals)

Other widely used urinary medications include analgesics,

such as Urobiotic (oxytetracycline hydrochloride, sulfamethizole, phenazopyridine hydrochloride); antispasmodics, such as Detrol Tablets (tolterodine tartrate); and parasympathomimetics, such as Urecholine (bethanechol chloride).

Vitamin and Mineral Supplements: Nutritionals SAFE

Vitamins, minerals, and other special nutritional preparations are **SAFE** for recovering alcoholics/addicts. This is true whether they are taken as therapy or for health maintenance. To be safe, take them on the basis of competent medical advice, and check their ingredients to be sure they contain no alcohol.

Contraceptives SAFE

Oral contraceptives for women, popularly called *birth control pills,* prevent pregnancy primarily by inhibiting ovulation. They are **SAFE** for recovering alcoholics/addicts.

Widely used birth control pills contain a progestin, a synthetic version of the female sex hormone progesterone. They include: the combined type, which also contains a natural or synthetic estrogen (such as Brevicon and Premarin); the progestogen-only type (such as Prometrium and Ovrette); and the phased-type, which contains varying proportions of a progestin and a natural or synthetic estrogen (for example, Ortho-Novum 10/11 21 and Triphasil-21).

Also **SAFE** for recovering alcoholics/addicts are various types of topical contraceptives applied locally within the vagina (such as spermicidal contraceptives in the form of creams, foams, and jellies); barrier contraceptives (such as diaphragms and condoms); and intrauterine devices implanted within the uterus.

Four

Safe Treatment for
Special Medical Conditions

Certain medical conditions can pose grave dangers of reactivating addiction for the recovering alcoholic/addict. These threats and ways of avoiding them are discussed in this chapter for

> pain, dental care,
> sleeplessness,
> hypertension, sexual disorders, smoking, eating disorders,
> mental illness, and
> chronic disease.

Pain

Dealing with pain as a recovering alcoholic/addict requires special effort and, on occasion, courage. Pain, of course, comes in many forms and in varying degrees, and every individual has a different threshold for tolerating it.

Alcoholics/addicts seem to focus more than others on physical discomfort. In fact, there is often an element of panic in the way recovering addicts react to mild or moderate pain. Such pain often provokes a desperate instinct in the alcoholic/addict to seek medication for relief without thinking clearly about the problem at hand. (Strangely enough, they often tolerate severe pain relatively well.)

First, it is necessary to emphasize the concept of cross-addiction. A recovering alcoholic still is in danger of activating the disease by using other mood-altering substances. He could either become addicted to the pain-relieving substance itself or be led back to his drug of choice, alcohol. Or at the very least, the individual could develop a dangerous habit of associating substances with a sense of physical or psychological relief.

Stan T., for instance, had been sober for five years when he developed chronic headaches. He had taken a drug called Fiorinal for headaches before he stopped drinking, and so he asked his doctor to renew the prescription. The doctor complied, and Stan began using Fiorinal tablets.

Soon both the headaches and the pill use increased. In time, it was difficult for Stan to know which was the prime problem—the headaches or the pills. Matters got worse, and Stan finally had to enter a hospital for detoxification.

Why did his tragic relapse occur? Well, Fiorinal contains a barbiturate (a sedative) that, for Stan, had become addicting. The drug also contains considerable amounts of caffeine, and as Stan's Fiornal abuse accelerated, many of his headaches could have been symptoms of caffeine withdrawal. Thus, Stan had felt he needed more pills, and the situation deteriorated. Stan's disease was activated, and denial reared its ugly head. Stan wouldn't accept the possibility that the pills could be a problem. He insisted that his only problem was "terrible headaches." That was his only focus.

Situations like Stan's are extremely complicated. They often confuse everybody for long periods of time. The disease of addiction will latch onto anything to nourish itself—and physical pain is one of those things. Then lies, deception, and denial can thrust a sober person into a costly, humiliating, and perhaps even fatal reactivation of the disease.

Caution therefore must accompany any type of pain treatment. Back problems, headaches, dental work, and minor injuries are some of the often minor ailments that may have major complications. Kathy M. comes to mind as another example. Kathy had been sober for three years when an old back problem was aggravated. The pain became quite severe, and at first, Kathy talked about it with her AA friends and merely rested and used heat treatments.

Soon, however, she grew quite depressed. She could do nothing but focus on the pain. She saw a doctor, who gave her a prescription for Tylenol with Codeine. She took the pills without discussing the move with her AA sponsor. Soon she was using them daily, and because of the pain, she stopped going to AA meetings. After several weeks she couldn't stop the pills, and she was still in pain. She was very depressed and began drinking.

Trials like these are very hard for the recovering alcoholic/addict. Pain, after all, is very real. In such situations, pain ruins the quality of life and interferes with the positive process of recovery. And significant pain leaves few alternatives to the use of mood-altering substances. What can recovering alcoholics/addicts do to safeguard continued abstinence? After all, they can't be expected to suffer unbearably. Here are some suggestions.

First, have any symptoms of pain evaluated medically. Learn as much as you can about the physical problem and therapeutic alternatives. Next, discuss the situation fully with your AA sponsor and others in the AA group. See what the experience of other members has been. If medication is necessary, make a plan with your sponsor.

We suggest that such a plan include the following actions:

1. Keep a written record of every dose of pain medication taken.
2. Call your sponsor before taking the medication.
3. Go to as many meetings as possible during this time, and talk about the situation there.
4. Discontinue the use of the medication as soon as possible.

Another technique might be to ask one's sponsor to keep the medicine so that a phone call is necessary to receive each dose. Of course, this is not always practical, but we know of situations where people went this far to protect their sobriety.

For those whose active addiction involved drugs, the management of pain is even more difficult. Although the same principles apply, for these addicts, exposure to pain-relieving narcotics has an even greater chance of triggering cravings and potential relapses.

Valerie M. used cocaine and Valium as well as alcohol. She eventually hit a horrible bottom, losing both her family and her job. She joined AA in terrible health and may not have survived much longer had she kept on drinking and drugging.

Valerie got sober with difficulty, but after a year and a half she was doing very well. She was working again, she had a cordial relationship with her former husband and her daughter, and she worked hard at her AA program. For the next four years, her recovery progressed. She helped many other recovering women, and life improved in all areas.

After six years of sobriety, severe headaches brought her to a doctor. Darvocet was prescribed, and Valerie took the pills without any special precautions, even though the doctor had told her they contained a narcotic. She went on using them for several weeks, and the headaches ceased. Valerie kept the pills in her medicine chest, but she didn't use them until a second siege of headaches occurred a month or so later.

A fellow AA member who saw Valerie take the pills registered surprise. Valerie said, "My doctor prescribed the medicine for my headache, and this kind of pill was never my thing anyhow." She went on periodically renewing the prescription and taking the pills for headaches as needed.

About a year later Valerie developed back pain, a flare-up of sciatica that had started after a horseback-riding accident twelve years before. She again began taking the Darvocet, but the back pain was so strong that the medicine didn't bring relief. Valerie didn't talk to people in AA about her distress. She went to several doctors, and got a prescription from one of them for Percodan. She knew this drug had a high potential for abuse, but she rationalized taking it, saying that narcotics were never "her thing" and besides the pain was so severe she had to take the Percodan.

Valerie tended to talk only to people who condoned her using the pills. When AA friends expressed concern, she avoided meetings. Soon she was taking pills every day and became obsessed with her pain. After many months of desperation, she was admitted to a hospital, and a long detoxification began. When Valerie left the hospital, she avoided AA meetings, began drinking, and is now in worse shape than when she first joined AA.

Valerie's case illustrates several principles. First, she used the initial medication without appropriate concern and safeguards. She took control of the medication herself and underplayed the danger. She began ignoring the reality of what she was doing and wouldn't listen to the warnings of her AA friends.

Next, Valerie took one of the most addictive euphoric narcotics, Percodan. Whether or not her back pain was severe, a red flag should have been raised at this point. Certain pain medications seem to be more addictive than others. Percodan is one. Dilaudid is another. Demerol is a third. All narcotics are addicting and thus dangerous for the recovering alcoholic/addict, but these three seem to be in a class by themselves: they are favored by active addicts and are treacherous therapy for alcoholics/addicts in recovery.

Another dimension to Valerie's case was her avoidance of meetings and AA friends who were disturbed by her drug use. When pain and drugs enter the life of a recovering alcoholic/addict, the disease gains incredible momentum. Denial and rationalization take over, and often the person begins manipulating everyone— AA friends, doctors, coworkers, and family. They remember that people say it's okay to take prescribed medications for a medical condition. They don't remember the cautions and restraints.

Stories like Valerie's vividly point out the need for the recovering alcoholic/addict to put decisions regarding pain treatment into the hands of AA colleagues and knowledgeable professionals. Use of pain-relieving drugs should never be left to the sole judgment of the recovering person. For normal people, the pain prescription often reads:

One or two tablets every four hours as needed for pain.

For alcoholics/addicts, it should read:

One dosage if absolutely necessary after fully discussing the need
for the medicine with your sponsor, and fully disclosing and
recording how many pills you have taken for this problem,
and seriously considering whether you can do without the pill,
and being aware and concerned about all properties, dangers, and
warnings with respect to this medication and your health.

Pain and drugs are a combination that any recovering alcoholic/ addict can never take too seriously or handle too carefully.

We must emphasize that other means of pain control should be considered and used instead of narcotics whenever possible. Among alternatives are physical therapies, acupuncture, biofeedback, and other techniques offered by specialized pain clinics or doctors. Although the recovering alcoholic/addict should evaluate such modalities carefully as to their applicability to his condition, he should not overlook them. It is always preferable that a recovering alcoholic/addict avoid mood-altering medications whenever possible. For example, if you have chronic pain, be sure to investigate local pain clinics. Some of them may offer techniques that you can substitute for medications, such as biofeedback.

Many nonnarcotic medications are safe for recovering alcoholics/addicts, including anti-inflammatory drugs such as Motrin, Advil, Naprosyn, and Indocin. It is true that these medications are rarely effective in completely relieving moderate to severe pain. However, for a recovering individual looking for safe alternatives to narcotics, these drugs in conjunction with physical techniques can often be used to manage even severe pain.

Pain management is a difficult challenge for a recovering alcoholic/addict. But when faced with pain, you should carefully consider the principles summarized here rather than resort to the careless use of prescription medications—use that could lead to a tragic loss of your sobriety.

Pain and Dental Care

Recovering alcoholics/addicts seem to want to take care of neglected teeth once their self-improvement program gets rolling. Many report having had a lot of dental problems during active substance abuse. Years of abuse may have had an effect on their teeth, and the ravages of nutritional deficiencies may have added to this damage.

Special hazards to continued abstinence posed by dental work include pain management and anesthesia. Nitrous oxide as a dental anesthetic should be avoided because it is a mood-altering substance. "Laughing gas," as nitrous oxide has long been called, is used as a recreational drug by some individuals. There are several alternatives for anesthesia, so recovering alcoholics/addicts should reject nitrous oxide whenever proposed.

Generally, dental work can be performed with local anesthetics, which are injected by hypodermic needle to numb the area being worked on. Such anesthetic agents (usually Xylocaine, a liquid anesthetic) are safe for people in recovery. They are sometimes mixed with epinephrine to lengthen their effect. Injections with added epinephrine give some people an uncomfortable sensation of overstimulation. However, the feeling passes in a short time. In general, for recovering alcoholics/addicts, local anesthesia is a safe alternative for blocking pain caused by dental work.

In addition, take care with pain medications that a dentist may give to relieve pain *after* dental work, especially extensive dental work. Be sure to follow the precautions set forth in the preceding pages.

Sleeplessness

Difficulty in falling asleep or staying asleep is often a problem early in sobriety. Certainly, insomnia is a common feature of detoxification or withdrawal. A simple principle applies if you have this problem: *No drugs should be used to help you sleep.*

Sleeplessness is surely an extremely uncomfortable state. But, as is often mentioned in recovery programs, no one ever dies from lack of sleep. When your body gets tired enough, sleep will come. During withdrawal, the body has to normalize. The effects of detoxification on the nervous system create an anxious, shaky, and often jittery state. Relaxation seems impossible.

Mild exercise such as a brisk walk during the day and a hot shower or bath at night often promote some degree of physical relaxation. However, if sleeplessness continues, you must simply bear it.

Once their early problems of insomnia pass, most recovering alcoholics/addicts have little difficulty with sleep. If periods of insomnia occur later in sobriety, again, drugs cannot be used. All sleeping pills are mood-altering—and some are especially dangerous for individuals in recovery.

Eddie P. had been sober for a year. He was doing well when a problem at work began to bother him. He became obsessed with something he considered unfair. Soon he couldn't sleep well, and he became irritable and more uncomfortable at work.

He talked about the work problem at his AA meetings and with his sponsor. But he never mentioned that he had seen his doctor about his insomnia, had obtained a prescription for a drug called Halcion, and had begun taking it at night. Soon he was using the pills almost every night and having difficulty sleeping when he didn't use them. His work problem passed, but the sleep problem persisted. Eddie began feeling tired and often took a Halcion pill upon getting home from work. He slept through several AA meetings and soon was attending meetings only occasionally.

Months later, he was still using the pills daily and had completely withdrawn from his AA activities. He became severely depressed, lost his job, and over a four-month period, lived isolated in his apartment. He then reached a bottom worse than the one that had originally brought him into AA.

Eventually, Eddie's brother alerted his AA friends to the sleeping-pill problem. An intervention was arranged, and ultimately Eddie entered a hospital program for detoxification. This was followed by a twenty-eight-day rehab. He eventually became sober again, but it was a rough trip. Eddie experienced the long-lasting mood swings that are characteristic of withdrawal from Halcion. Halcion and similar drugs can cause depression for months after their use is discontinued.

Many cases of sleeping-pill addiction develop among addiction-prone individuals. In view of this, the principle for the recovering alcoholic/addict is rigid: do not take any medications for sleeplessness.

Associated Diseases

Certain diseases and compulsive habits are frequently associated with alcoholism. Some of these problems result from the physical effects of alcohol, and some from the accompanying psychological and emotional dysfunction.

HYPERTENSION

Hypertension, or high blood pressure, is medically important because, if left untreated, it hastens the development of athero-sclerotic cardiovascular disease and related problems. High blood pressure is linked to strokes, heart attacks, and other medical problems related to blood-vessel abnormalities.

Alcoholics have several problems related to hypertension. For one, alcohol itself affects blood pressure. When one is drinking, intoxication and withdrawal constantly fluctuate. Both states stress the cardiovascular system and can produce hypertension.

Often, when alcoholics are seen medically during their years of drinking, they are found to be hypertensive. They may receive medication for high blood pressure, and then upon becoming sober, they assume the medication is still necessary. Indeed, it might not be. In other words, a diagnosis of hypertension made during active drinking is unreliable. On getting sober, an alcoholic with a history of hypertension should consult a physician for a blood pressure reevaluation. Medications that were previously prescribed might not be needed after sobriety is established.

This evaluation should not be undertaken too soon, however, for blood pressure during withdrawal and detoxification is unstable and often elevated. This period of time is best monitored by a physician for a variety of reasons. However, an evaluation for hypertension should be repeated after the period of withdrawal is complete. The history of Jim W. is illustrative. Jim was a school principal whose drinking was a problem for more than twenty years. During that time he saw different physicians for various problems. At one point he was told he had high blood pressure, measured at 160/110.

Several medicines were tried in an attempt to treat his hypertension, and eventually he was stabilized on a drug called Inderal. After this medication had been started, Jim saw other physicians, all of whom legitimately kept him on the Inderal.

Jim began his sobriety in a well-known alcohol rehabilitation center and proceeded to do well. During his early sobriety, he came to the author's office for a problem of impotency. This condition had been bothering him for years, but during his drinking, he neither cared enough nor was functional enough to engage in sexual activity.

After assessing the impotency problem, it seemed there were two issues at hand. First, the drug Inderal can cause impotency. And second, Jim's blood pressure was now 130/70 on the medication. Since Jim was in good health otherwise, the author decided to test two hypotheses by stopping the Inderal. First, we would see whether Jim's impotency was related to the medication. Second, we would find out whether Jim's hypertension was due to the effects of his drinking.

As it turned out, Jim's blood pressure remained normal with no medication. He had no underlying hypertension after all. Then, after a short time, sexual function returned.

Many medical patterns, especially hypertension, are brought on during active alcohol and drug use and may or may not continue after normalization of the body in sobriety. Of course, an alcoholic may have real hypertension. One should not stop medication upon attaining sobriety without an evaluation by a doctor.

SEXUAL DISORDERS

Jim W.'s sexual problem brought his unnecessary treatment for blood pressure to light. In this situation, medication was the major cause of his impotency. However, Jim's sexual problem was not only physical.

As mentioned earlier, throughout his years of drinking, Jim had no active sexual functioning. The medication may have been part of the reason for his decreased libido, but other factors certainly played a role as well. Jim was married throughout his drinking years. His wife, over the last ten years of his drinking, had become angry and uncommunicative. She resented his unreliable, self-centered behavior. She felt no warmth toward him and had no desire to pursue a sexual relationship.

Jim's daily life involved a pattern of coming home from work, drinking himself into a stupor, and either passing out in front of the television or dragging himself to bed. He had no room for any relationship, sexual or personal. Alcoholism had filled every pore of his personality. When not intoxicated, Jim admitted to having felt both disgusted with himself and sexually inadequate.

His sexual problem had many facets. There was lack of libido. There was a deteriorating, and ultimately disastrous, personal relationship with his wife due to his alcoholic behavior. There was in Jim a feeling of self-disgust and a total personality disintegration. Obviously, a sexual relationship could not survive.

His scenario is typical. Active alcoholics/addicts can rarely sustain healthy sexual relationships. Their sexual problems run the gamut from physical to emotional and reflect the inability of interpersonal relationships to survive in a climate of active addiction.

Couples afflicted by active addiction of one or both members often stay together because of other needs, such as emotional dependency, financial support, family cohesion, religious compliance, or outward respectability. But the basis is seldom healthy sexual and personal fulfillment.

As a result, when recovery begins, sexual problems often need attention. As the alcoholic/addict develops in early recovery, he or she must face the destructive effect of the disease on interpersonal relationships. Certainly, normal sexual activity doesn't develop immediately on cessation of drinking.

Through the AA program, the recovering individual gradually learns to act in a responsible and mature manner with regard to close relationships. Intimate relationships such as marriage can often be restored to a fulfilling and healthy state, and a good sexual relationship can be part of this change. However, the process may take a long time—years, in some cases.

The sexual disorders reported by men and women in recovery usually relate to libido and male impotence. Margaret T., for example, was seen by the author during an outpatient detoxification program. During this time, she expressed the sense of feeling "neuter." She had no desire for sexual contact. She also lived an isolated existence working as a private-duty nurse at night, and coming home to sleep in her apartment during the day.

As Margaret progressed in her sobriety, she became more concerned with her lifestyle. She saw the limitations of her isolation, and although she didn't feel any return of sexual desire, she did discover in herself a need for social contact. Soon it became apparent that her job was confining, and she took a position as an office nurse, working in the daytime. She gradually made friends but was afraid to date and was concerned about her lack of sexual desire.

Although AA helped Margaret to grow as a person, she sought private counseling as well. She soon became aware that social life and interpersonal relationships were important to her and were missing from her life because of alcoholism. She took steps to change. After some months her life took on a more normal pattern. She began dating, and after eighteen months of sobriety, Margaret had a successful sexual relationship. Her life now has the usual ups and downs, but she has normal sexual function and a healthy social life.

The point here is that sexual problems are not isolated disorders, but are intricately related to the entire disease of alcoholism or addiction. As recovery progresses and the emotional ravages of the disease of addiction lift, sexual problems generally dissipate. There may be some problems that require more specific therapy, but, in general, patience will be rewarded.

Sexual disorders don't affect every alcoholic, but the prevalence of sexual problems among alcoholics/addicts is high. The emotional and psychological aspects of the disease combine with the physical effects of alcohol or drugs. Alcohol, for example, affect the blood vessels, the liver (which metabolizes many hormones), and the central nervous system, all of which are involved in the sexual response. Cocaine, in particular, has extremely debilitating effects on the sexual response. All drugs must be cleared from the system, and a significant period of time must pass for the physiological component of the sexual response to normalize.

Men find their most frequent pattern of sexual difficulty to be indifference and impotence as the later stages of alcoholism are reached. Frank P., for instance, was married, and as his alcoholism progressed, his wife could not relate sexually to him. Frank sought relationships outside the marriage. After two years of promiscuity, though, he became less interested in sexual activity, and on the few occasions when he did become involved sexually, he experienced impotency. This intensified his growing self-disgust and feelings of inadequacy. By the end of his active drinking, Frank gave up even trying to perform sexually. He had little desire and feared sexual failure.

Frank's case is an example of the complex issues that develop in addiction. A disintegrating marital relationship, destructive promiscuity, sexual failures, and avoidance of sexual activity are all part of a common pattern. With the advent of sobriety, there is usually a restoration of a more normal sex life. However, first the alcoholic/addict must begin recovery step by step, slowly healing wounds and reconstructing his or her personality, feelings, and relationships.

As this recovery matures, sexual attitudes and function return to a more normal state. Recovery doesn't guarantee sexual health. For some, problems linger, and others need professional help—but so do nonalcoholics. As in most areas, honesty, proceeding with the basic AA principles of recovery, and patience will yield rewarding results.

Finally, it should be noted that many recovering alcoholics/addicts are also the children of alcoholics/addicts, a group that has suffered a higher than normal incidence of sexual abuse in childhood. Sexual dysfunction in recovery for those with a history of such abuse might result in part from repressed painful experiences. In cases like this, normal sexual function might be restored if these experiences are dealt with in therapy conducted by a qualified professional.

SMOKING

Many members who smoke, and a coffee urn or two, are typical hallmarks of an AA meeting. The message is clear: alcoholics smoke a lot, and they drink a lot of coffee. Because they are addiction-prone, these predilections are not surprising. Nicotine and caffeine are drugs prevalent in our society. Of course, addicts will succumb in greater proportion than nonaddicts.

It has been a longtime principle among alcohol treatment programs to consider smoking a necessary evil for the nicotine-addicted recovering alcoholic. To ask the alcoholic who smokes to give up a second addiction is just too much. However, in recent years, the evidence demonstrating the ill effects of tobacco has been widely publicized. Medical studies indicate that respiratory problems and illnesses, as well as cancer and heart disease, are more prevalent among smokers than nonsmokers.

Consequently, attitudes are changing. Many treatment programs, AA included, now have nonsmoking meetings. The alcoholic might do well not to rely on the enabling principle that to cease smoking during early recovery causes too much stress and is too distracting. For some, it may be, but the health issues at hand demand a new attitude. Smoking is too dangerous—perhaps even to people around the smoker—not to be confronted as unhealthy and worth stopping by the recovering alcoholic.

On the other hand, sobriety still must come first, because alcoholism/addiction is the more urgently dangerous compulsion. Moreover, a recovering alcoholic/addict who slips is very unlikely to stop smoking. For reasons like these, sponsors in AA often advise a person who wants to stop smoking to wait until after the first year of sobriety. Individuals thus well established in abstinence frequently find that the practices and social support of AA that worked for their drink/drug compulsion also prove effective against their smoking addiction.

EATING DISORDERS

The compulsive disorder that allows alcoholism or addiction to flourish may also be manifested by other unhealthy behavior. Smoking is one example; excessive coffee drinking is another. Eating disorders, as a group, also exemplify maladaptive behavior rooted in the same compulsive drives that fuel addiction.

We should not assume that these compulsive disorders overlap, but they are seen in the alcoholic population with more than average frequency. Certainly there are nonalcoholic smokers, overeaters, anorexics, and other types of compulsives, and certainly many alcoholics are spared these problems. Nevertheless, among alcoholics/addicts, relatively few have been completely free of at least one of these associated compulsions.

When first entering recovery, individuals with these compulsions usually find them operating in full force. It is often advised that sobriety be stabilized before any attempt is made to discontinue other compulsive habits. This theory assumes that all energies are needed for efforts related to achieving comfortable sobriety. It is often suggested that one wait before attacking smoking, overeating, or other compulsions than alcohol/drug abuse. Such suggestions constructively counter the frequent but unwise eagerness of the newly sober person to cure everything at once. Putting "first things first," in the words of the familiar AA slogan, is instead commonly and properly advised.

Eating disorders constitute a group of complex compulsive patterns of behavior. Overeating with resulting obesity is probably the most common. Anorexia and bulimia are two other disorders. Many alcoholics begin recovery having neglected their health in general, but particularly in the realm of nutrition. Compulsive overeating can sometimes flare up in early recovery. The overweight person who is in early recovery and is a compulsive overeater has few tools to use in regard to his or her eating disorder.

Concentration is on the principles of recovery, and these principles are not integrated enough into the recovering individual's personality and behavior to be generalized to other areas of living. Compulsive overeaters often gain weight during early recovery. Although this is distressing, patience is advisable. Fad diets and extreme measures to deal with obesity are particularly unhealthy at this time.

Eventually, as the anxieties of everyday living are more naturally handled using the principles of recovery programs, and as moods are somewhat stabilized, the compulsive eating is more easily controlled.

In dealing with drinking or drugs, abstinence is the foundation of recovery. The first drink or drug will ruin sobriety and trigger eventual relapse. With overeating, abstinence is obviously not the answer. However, one can correlate any compulsive eating with a first drink. If the alcoholic is powerless over alcohol, as an overeater he can think of himself as powerless over compulsive eating. Thus, a three-meal-a-day, nutritionally balanced, moderate- calorie intake can be positively and safely established. The first time the overeater grabs a handful of cookies or otherwise lets go and eats because of a compulsive drive, he or she is probably in for a damaging food-binge slip. Many obese compulsive overeaters who are recovering from alcoholism/addiction can use the principles of the recovery program to replace their other compulsions with healthy behavior.

However, this takes time. It seems to be after the second or third year of recovery that many overeaters or anorexics and bulimics begin to deal with their eating disorders successfully. These disorders have lifelong roots and emotionally charged associations. Therefore patience, honesty about one's feelings, and steady progress in sobriety usually produce success with eating disorders in recovering alcoholics/addicts. Some alcoholics/addicts with deep-seated and stubborn cases of anorexia and bulimia find that special medical or psychotherapeutic treatment, or both, also helps to deal with the disorders.

Mental Illness

At least in part, alcoholism itself qualifies as a mental illness. A classic view in the field is expressed in the core sourcebook of

AA, *Alcoholics Anonymous,* which holds that alcoholism is a three-fold disease having physical, mental, and spiritual components. (It also sets forth a second step of recovery involving action by alcoholics "to restore us to sanity.") Moreover, the official diagnostic manual of the American Psychiatric Association defines the symptoms of alcohol or drug dependence as a mental illness.

Mental illness—or the possibility of mental illness—complicates alcoholism/addiction and recovery from it in two respects that have far-reaching implications.

First, what often masquerades as a separate mental illness (e.g., depression) before recovery, turns out in recovery to have been primarily the disease of alcoholism/addiction. The misdiagnosis is frequently made by the alcoholic/addict and by his or her psychiatrist as well. This is especially true with anxiety and depression. Anxiety, depression, and other psychiatric manifestations of alcoholism/addiction generally subside as the process of recovery strengthens.

Second, some persons who are alcoholics/addicts also suffer from an additional psychiatric disorder or mental illness. In such cases, their recovery (through total abstinence and progress in a recovery program such as AA or NA) does not alone relieve the second emotional disorder or mental illness. Guidelines based on experience can help you decide in the face of psychiatric symptoms on the most effective ways to assure safety and promote recovery from both afflictions.

GUIDELINES FOR DEALING WITH MENTAL ILLNESS *AND* ALCOHOLISM/ADDICTION

If you are a recovering alcoholic/addict and think you may have a mental illness in addition to alcoholism/addiction, you should follow a number of guidelines for health and safety. These guidelines reflect a consensus of wide clinical experience as well as experience gained by those in recovery.

1. IF NECESSARY, TAKE IMMEDIATE EMERGENCY ACTION FOR SAFETY

If you are a recovering alcoholic/addict and are feeling suicidal— or if an active or recovering alcoholic/addict close to you is talking about committing suicide—get immediate help from a psychiatrist, possibly by going to a hospital emergency room. Moreover, police respond to calls involving suicide attempts. Suicidal feelings and attempts are not uncommon among active alcoholics/addicts, especially when they become sickened and desperate because of their disease and are nearing their bottom.

If a family member with alcoholism/addiction has violent outbreaks, seek immediate help. Call the police. They should take the individual to the emergency room of a hospital for diagnosis. This also applies if you yourself are an alcoholic/addict in recovery and are having uncontrollable outbreaks of violence that worry you after they've passed. If so, you should act immediately on the next guideline.

2. GET AND FOLLOW THE ADVICE OF A PSYCHIATRIST WELL INFORMED ABOUT ALCOHOLISM/ADDICTION

When you first see in yourself as a recovering alcoholic/addict (or in a family member who is recovering) evidence of a disorder or mental illness besides alcoholism/addiction, consult a psychiatrist well informed about alcoholism/addiction. Don't act as a doctor yourself in deciding what the condition is. Also, don't let anyone else act as the doctor. Get and follow the psychiatrist's diagnosis and recommendation for treatment.

If you are an alcoholic/addict and actively participate in a recovery program, talk over what you're doing for a mental illness and why with your sponsor (and possibly with other friends in the program). They should approve of this course of yours if they're experienced and informed. For instance, according to the official AA pamphlet, *The AA Member: Medications and Other Drugs,* "No AA member plays doctor."

Also, follow this book's advice about working with doctors, including psychiatrists. Be sure to observe three stipulations: choose a psychiatrist thoroughly informed about alcoholics/addicts and recovery; be absolutely honest with the doctor about your alcoholism/ addiction; and if a medication is prescribed, make sure to take it only in the dosages and at the intervals prescribed.

In addition, be wary of recommendations that you use any minor tranquilizer, sedative, psychostimulant, or narcotic drug. As explained in chapter three, these drugs are dangerous to recovering alcoholics/addicts because of the risk of reactivating acute alcohol or drug abuse. Should such drugs be proposed for you, ask the psychiatrist if a medication safe for alcoholics/addicts might be substituted.

If a "safe" medication cannot be substituted, follow all the precautions for drugs dangerous to alcoholics/addicts discussed earlier in this chapter and in chapter three. Also, ask the psychiatrist to lower the dosage and stop the medication if—and as soon as—it is feasible to do so.

Getting—and following—competent psychiatric advice without delay can prove critically important. This is illustrated by a particularly unfortunate case.

Stan B. felt the depression from which he had long suffered grow deeper and deeper after he had been sober and active in AA for seven months. The depression had lifted somewhat when he'd first started recovery and the depressant effects of alcohol had dissipated. But the depression had then returned worse than ever before. Neither at that time nor before had he obtained a psychiatric evaluation and recommendation for treating his depression.

Stan never admitted to his AA sponsor and friends that he felt much worse than before. As a result, he never learned that other members of his group had also felt hideously depressed and had found relief through psychiatric treatment. Some afflicted with clinical depression had been helped by antidepressant medications, which are nonaddictive. Others who suffered extreme mood swings (bipolar illness) were on carefully worked-out doses of lithium carbonate, also nonaddictive, which had largely stabilized their moods. And in particular, Stan had never learned that before getting medications, these fellow AA members had also been tormented by thoughts of suicide.

One weekend Stan phoned his sponsor to say he was feeling terrible and was afraid of what he might do. His sponsor rushed to Stan's house but arrived too late. Stan had already left in his car and had driven at high speed on a local highway, ramming into a tree and killing himself.

3. BEGIN RECOVERY FROM ALCOHOLISM/ADDICTION (OR GET YOUR FAMILY MEMBER STARTED)

It may be that you're already being treated for a mental illness diagnosed by a psychiatrist, and you also know that you suffer from alcoholism/addiction as well. If this is true, make every effort to start recovery. Join an AA or NA group, and try to go to meetings daily for three months. Follow all actions suggested to help you become an active and committed member. Or, if you need to begin as an inpatient or outpatient going through rehabilitation (possibly preceded by detoxification), by all means do that, and then become active in AA or NA.

After your first three months, continue working hard at

recovering. You may find that the program helps substantially to relieve the mental illness you have.

In the case of a family member, try to persuade him or her to follow this advice. That is, if the family member is being treated for a mental illness but is also an alcoholic/addict, urge him or her to enter a recovery program.

4. RECOVERY FROM MENTAL ILLNESS MAY BE IMPEDED UNLESS RECOVERY FROM ALCOHOLISM/ADDICTION IS BEGUN

Progress in recovering from a mental illness may be slowed or blocked entirely if you are an alcoholic/addict and you do not get started in recovery. Tom R., for instance, was a diagnosed schizophrenic who heard voices. At times, he thought he was the illegitimate son of God and could ask God to take away all the nuclear bombs from the earth on a spaceship and keep them safely in another galaxy. He was also multiply addicted, mainly abusing alcohol, marijuana, cocaine, and LSD.

Tom was treated by a psychiatrist for nine years and was kept sedated by heavy doses of Thorazine and Prolixin. They stabilized his schizophrenia, but there was little or no improvement over the years, and his alcoholism/addiction continued unchecked. For most of those years he was completely unemployable and lived on welfare. Because of his alcoholism, he had three DWI convictions and was convicted as well for driving without a license. He was thus facing a felony sentence of up to four years in jail.

Tom's judge said that if Tom spent six months in an alcoholism recovery program, he wouldn't have to go to jail (though he would serve an overall five-year suspended sentence under tight control of his parole officer). So Tom entered a six-week inpatient alcoholism program at a state psychiatric hospital and continued in an outpatient day program for alcoholism over the rest of the six months. At the same time he was as active as he could be in AA. His schizophrenia improved markedly after he progressed in abstinence and sobriety. He could live independently and hold jobs while being maintained on relatively light and decreasing doses of Thorazine.

A report to the U.S. Congress in 2002 stated that "about 51 percent of those [persons] with one or more lifetime mental disorders also have a lifetime history of at least one substance abuse disorder." This annual report to the Congress was made by the federal agency SAMHSA. In all, it noted, seven million to ten million Americans suffer or have suffered from both mental illness and alcoholism/addiction. This is more than half of all Americans who develop mental illness.

"From studies and first-hand experience," the report also notes, "many researchers and clinicians believe that both disorders must be addressed as primary and treated as such." Of course, taking both to be primary means that ignoring the alcoholism/addiction while providing treatment only to relieve the mental illness will bring little or no improvement in mental health.

"Sometimes the chemical dependency is paramount, and you can't get to the psychiatric disorder until you come to grips with the addiction," the head of the addictive disorders services at the Mayo Clinic once remarked in this connection.

Our opinion is that this is true not only for psychiatric disorders, but for problems of many other kinds. That is, persons suffering from alcoholism/addiction can make little or no progress on such other problems as marital relations, sexual dysfunction, weight, or even elevated blood-pressure problems until they begin a program of recovery from the alcoholism/addiction.

5. AFTER LONG PROGRESS IN RECOVERY, REASSESS THE DIAGNOSIS AND TREATMENT, AND ADJUST ACCORDINGLY

Each year of active participation in AA or NA with complete abstinence from alcohol and any other former drugs of choice, you and your psychiatrist should reassess the diagnosis and treatment plan for your mental illness. On one of these annual reviews, you may find that the mental illness has begun clearing up, possibly to the point of enabling you to plan with your psychiatrist a careful tryout sequence of reducing your medication. You may even find that treatment might be tentatively brought to an end in the near future.

For instance, Harriet L. had experienced episodes of intense rage and intense depression after starting to recover from her alcoholism. After some eight months in AA, she found that these episodes had become much less frequent and upsetting. But then her mother died, and in a few weeks her depression returned with its old intensity. She tried the AA methods that had worked before to ease her depression, such as phoning her sponsor when feeling troubled and attending more meetings. But most of the time they failed to bring relief. Some mornings she was so depressed that she couldn't get out of bed and couldn't even phone anyone.

Her sponsor stopped by on one of these occasions when the depression was making Harriet feel completely helpless and hopeless. The sponsor suggested that Harriet should see a psychiatrist who had helped some other members of their AA group. Harriet was soon put on an antidepressant medication and began seeing the psychiatrist for therapy twice a week. Harriet's mother had been extremely harsh, brutal, cold, and domineering. Harriet was able to bring her long-stifled and agonized feelings about her mother to light in the therapy sessions. And the medication seemed to lift that black, immobilizing despair of her depression.

After about eighteen months of therapy, Harriet no longer fell prey to bouts of deep depression and felt far more at peace with and knowledgable about what had really happened between her and her mother. She and the psychiatrist decided to try one therapy session a week and to gradually reduce the medication. After about six months, Harriet felt even better. She and the psychiatrist decided on a trial ending of both therapy sessions and medication. Since then, Harriet has not felt depressed.

Chronic Disease

Sobriety guarantees a quality of life that gradually improves in all dimensions. However, difficulties, tragedy, disease, and misfortune are part of any life, even a sober one. The alcoholic who had lost, or failed to develop, adequate coping skills while actively drinking learns in sobriety to deal with life's hardships without drinking. Recovery programs give the alcoholic/addict tools to deal with the ups and the downs.

Chronic disease is difficult for anyone to handle. Most people when confronted with a chronic disease react first with disbelief and later with anger, depression, and acceptance. Recovering alcoholics/ addicts must go through the same emotions when they fall victim to chronic disease.

There are two major considerations for recovering alcoholics/ addicts afflicted with chronic disease. One is that care must be exercised in dealing with pain (see "Pain" earlier in this chapter). The second is that they should accept the help offered by the programs and people of AA and related organizations.

ARTHRITIS

Clark B. was sober for two years when he developed severe joint pains and a general sense of fatigue. His doctor performed a number of tests and discovered that Clark had rheumatoid arthritis. The doctor told Clark that although the disease had a variable course, he could expect to deal with chronic pain and stiffness.

At first, Clark denied the reality of a long-term disability, but when his joints continued to hurt and his energy remained low, he became quite depressed. Fortunately, his physician knew the principles of recovery and did not offer Clark pain medication. However, he did prescribe anti-inflammatory drugs and a course of steroid therapy (see "Corticosteroids" in chapter three). Clark's energy increased and his pain lessened, but when the medication was stopped, the pain increased.

When Clark had to give up his job as a carpenter, he became even more depressed. He was withdrawn for a few months, attending few AA meetings and never sharing his feelings. His mood gradually became more bleak.

One day, at the urging of his AA sponsor, Clark went to a meeting and discussed his fears and anxieties with his group. The outpouring of understanding and support made Clark feel better. He began to participate more actively in his recovery program, and he steadily gained strength. Soon he accepted his illness and coped adequately. Eventually, he obtained an office job in construction accounting work. Overall, he has been managing well, though he has to cope with intermittent pain.

Clark's story illustrates the therapeutic effect a recovery program can have. Both his mood and his pain improved when he used the tools of AA.

Rheumatoid arthritis is one of the most aggressive and painful types of arthritis. The more common osteoarthritis—typical age-associated arthritis—can be quite painful as well.

Medications safe for recovering alcoholics/addicts can help with arthritic pain, but strong analgesics must be avoided except in special circumstances (see "Pain" in this chapter). Among other methods of dealing with arthritic pain are physical therapy, low-impact exercise (swimming, for example), and biofeedback.

DIABETES

Another not uncommon chronic disease is *diabetes mellitus*. Probably its best known feature is a relative lack of the body's naturally produced hormone insulin, and the body's resulting difficulty in controlling the blood sugar level. As this disease progresses, it can affect the cardiovascular system, kidneys, and other organs.

Dietary measures and careful control of blood sugar through insulin injections can minimize the progress of diabetes. But it remains a chronic disease that requires lifelong attention. Because lifestyle habits such as eating, weight control, and exercise must be modified in order to control diabetes, the recovering alcoholic/addict has to deal with such difficult issues as impulse control, discipline, and giving up certain pleasures.

Again, there are no easy solutions. Diabetics are dealing with a chronic disease requiring behavior modification. Therefore, recovering alcoholics/addicts who are diabetic should fully use their recovery program. Fear, anger, depression, and anxiety are all part of dealing with a chronic disease—and diabetes, as pointed out, has inherent problems. AA and similar programs offer the alcoholic/addict a means of dealing with these emotions, emotions that battle against sobriety. Recovering alcoholics/addicts with diabetes must exercise their greatest maturity and coping abilities to deal with their two diseases concurrently.

HEART DISEASE

Heart disease is common in almost all populations. The most common form is coronary artery disease, in which the blood vessels feeding the heart muscle are obstructed. Types of heart disease related to coronary artery disease include myocardial infarctions (or heart attacks), congestive heart failure, certain cardiac rhythm disturbances, and angina.

For recovering alcoholics/addicts, the same principles apply to heart disease as to other chronic diseases. At the onset of heart disease, negative emotions are strong, and if sobriety is not strong as well, a relapse into active addiction, or at least into "dry drunk" emotional misery, can result.

With heart disease, a sense of vulnerability and doom typically begins a period of depression, fear, and a sense of inadequacy. These emotions are dangerous for the alcoholic/addict. Only recovery-program principles and the support of these programs can ensure adequate coping with a difficult time of life.

Most heart medications are without reactivation risk for the alcoholic/addict.

CANCER

Cancer has an emotional impact unlike that of any other disease. Although in reality cancer is many different diseases with many different outcomes, when people learn they have cancer, they usually react with fear and a sense of doom. Everyone, alcoholic or not, can use help and support when first diagnosed with cancer. The recovering alcoholic/addict has to be particularly careful with some of the attitudes or reflexes that are part of the disease of addiction.

Negativism and projection (needless worry about future outcomes) are two tendencies that certainly might emerge here. To some degree, this is one time that such feelings might be normal. The alcoholic/addict, however, needs to guard against letting these attitudes and feelings become excessive and damaging. The best way to ensure against a flare-up of alcoholic attitudes is to intensify contact with the recovery program. Group support is particularly beneficial at times of crisis, offering a perspective that is often extremely valuable. An alcoholic who deals with cancer alone is bound to experience more pain than if he or she accepts the help offered by his fellow alcoholics/addicts.

By discussing their fears with the recovery group, alcoholics/addicts are bound to find others who have had similar problems. They will learn that cancer has many potential outcomes, not just those they fearfully project. (In fact, today treatment for cancer can prove effective, and in many cases, a cure is likely.) Expressing feelings is helpful in itself. Conversely, alcoholics/addicts who keep their problem to themselves and withdraw will probably see their alcoholic attitudes grow, giving them two active diseases to deal with. They may despair and face the danger of drinking or drugging—a course that would tragically undercut their most essential personal resources.

An alcoholic/addict afflicted with a type of cancer that leads to advanced disease faces one of the more difficult situations life has to offer. Numerous experiences have shown that the principles and support of one's alcoholism/addiction recovery program can also be valuable in situations like this. Here, alcoholics/addicts may confront the problem of dealing with narcotic pain relievers. There are no universally right answers in this difficult area. In our experience, however, alcoholics/addicts can safely take these medications for real pain arising in such situations.

Appendix:

SOURCES OF
INFORMATION AND HELP

This appendix provides sources of information beyond that given in this book, and information that will help you carry out actions suggested herein. With these sources, you can obtain further information on

- narcotic controlled substances, often used medically to relieve acute pain but illegal in the United States unless prescribed,
- prescription and nonprescription medications of all kinds, and highly detailed information about them,
- physicians certified in the treatment of alcoholism/ addiction,
- and current research on alcoholism/addiction.

You can also consult these sources for help with

- finding alcoholism/addiction treatment centers and programs, that can refer you to physicians who fully understand the affliction,

- and finding local groups of major self-help recovery organizations, groups possibly beneficial to you for information, advice, and moral support.

Narcotic Controlled Substances

Highly addictive substances are illegal in the United States unless prescribed by certain licensed medical professionals for officially specified therapeutic purposes, and dispensed by licensed pharmacists. Both the medical professional and the pharmacist must adhere to strictly enforced recording requirements.

Among these substances are powerful drugs for relieving acute pain. Their use is tightly controlled because of the high probability that normal people taking them will become addicted. In fact, the U.S. statute making them illegal identifies them in Schedules I, II, III, IV, and V, ranging from the most highly and dangerously addictive in Schedule I, to those of lowest addicting potential in Schedule V.

While these substances are officially deemed very dangerous to normal individuals, they are even more dangerous to women and men recovering from alcoholism/addiction. For them, it is crucial to know what these substances are, and what precautions to take should a medical need make taking them imperative.

Safe Medicines for Sober People provides just such information. However, a reader who wants to see the full list of federally controlled substances may look it up in the Comprehensive Drug Abuse Prevention and Control Act of 1970 and its amendments. One convenient way to do so is by going to the following Web site: www4.law.cornell.edu/uscode/21/812.html. Click on "Sec.812.— Schedules of controlled substances." There you will find definitions of the five schedules, and a list of the substances in each schedule.

The substances are identified by their main chemical names. Ones you might recognize include, in Schedule I, Codeine Methylbromide, Heroin, Morphine Methylbromide, "Marihuana" [sic], Mescaline, and Peyote.

Prescription and Nonprescription Medications

Additional information on medications that this book discusses can be found in reference volumes and on the Internet.

REFERENCE BOOKS

Physicians' Desk Reference (Medical Economics Co., ed., Montvale, NJ: Medical Economics Co.). Familiarly called the *PDR,* each annual edition of this work runs more than three thousand pages. For each of thousands of medications, it presents the extensive prescribing information approved by the U.S. Food and Drug Administration (FDA). This is the same highly detailed information that you get in leaflet form when you pick up a prescription drug from a pharmacy. Indexes in the *PDR,* especially one by brand name and generic name for individual drugs, make the book easy to use.

Medical Economics Company also publishes a number of related works in book or CD form, including *Physicians' Desk Reference for Nonprescription Drugs and Dietary Supplements.* Its annual editions are a major source for nonprescription drug information.

Detailed information about each work in the *PDR* family can be found at www.PDRbookstore.com.

Extensive and authoritative information on individual medications can be found in the annual volumes of the "United States

Pharmacopeia Dispensing Information" series (identified by the registered trademark "USP DI"). These books are primarily professional reference works and are held by many libraries. The ones most likely to interest readers of *Safe Medicine for Sober People* are as follows.

USP DI Drug Reference Guides, Volume I: Drug Information for the Health-Care Professional and *Volume II: Advice for the Patient* (United States Pharmacopeial Convention, Inc., ed., Thomson Micromedex).

Further information about these works is available at www.micromedex.com/products/uspdi.

WEB SITES

Although many Web sites provide data on medications, one in particular provides authoritative, extensive, and up-to-date information: http://medlineplus.gov, "the world's largest medical library."

On the medline homepage, click on Drug Information. You will then be able to search for detailed information on individual medications.

Physicians Certified in Alcoholism/Addiction Treatment

The American Society of Addiction Medicine and the American Academy of Addiction Psychiatry offer certification of physicians in the diagnosis and treatment of alcoholism/addiction, as explained in chapter two. Neither association provides the names of certified physicians.

However, such a service is provided by the American Medical Association through its Web site: www.ama-assn.org. Once you access the AMA homepage, click on Patients-Go. Then click on Doctor Finder. You will then see a screen for the AMA Physician Select service. You can then enter the cities or towns in which you want to find certified physicians, as well as the area of certification you are seeking.

Treatment Centers and Physician Referrals

Centers and programs that provide treatment for alcoholism/addiction will often be able to recommend doctors who are knowledgeable about the disease. To find nearby treatment centers and programs, you can access a national directory of more than 11,000 such treatment facilities by going to http://findtreatment.samhsa.gov.

Referrals to alcoholism/addiction treatment facilities are also available from a hotline service operated by the U.S. government. Its toll-free number is: 1-800-729-6686.

Self-Help Recovery Organizations

Members of local groups of major self-help recovery organizations should be able to recommend doctors who are knowledgeable about alcoholism/addiction. There are several ways to find nearby groups of AA.

In the United States, look in the local phone directory to reach AA. You'll find AA and/or Alcoholics Anonymous listed in the directory's white pages, or in the yellow pages, under a heading like Alcoholism Information and Treatment Centers. Local police also can often tell you where and when nearby AA meetings are held.

Outside the United States, you can similarly try local phone directories. You can also use the telephone numbers, mailing address, and Web site discussed in the following paragraphs.

Another way to find local AA groups is to contact Alcoholics Anonymous World Services, Inc. This is the AA General Service Office for the United States and Canada, as well as the publisher of official AA literature and coordinator of AA worldwide. Its mailing address is P.O. Box 459, New York, NY 10163, and its phone number is 212-870-3400. You can also reach it through its Web site: www.aa.org.

This site has links to AA "intergroup" telephone information services for many metropolitan areas and regions of the United States and Canada. AA intergroup services have detailed information on local AA groups and their meetings in the intergroup area.

You can find local groups and central offices of Narcotics Anonymous (NA) and Cocaine Anonymous (CA) as follows: Groups of NA or CA in your area might be listed in the local telephone directory. However, it might be more effective to contact the NA or CA central offices.

Narcotics Anonymous World Service, P.O. Box 9999, Van Nuys, CA 91409. Telephone: 818-773-9999. Web site: www.na.org

Cocaine Anonymous World Services Office, P.O. Box 2000, Los Angeles, CA 90049-8000. Telephone: 310-559-5833. Web site: www.ca.org

Research on Alcoholism/Addiction

To learn of current research developments in alcoholism/addiction, consult the sources given in this section. Those presented represent a number of major sources, but by no means all of them.

Two leading scholarly periodicals in the field are issued by professional societies and are published quarterly.

Journal of Addictive Diseases. Published by the American Society of Addictive Medicine, 4601 North Park Ave., Arcade Suite

101, Chevy Chase, MD 20815. Telephone: 301-656-3920. Web site: www.asam.org.

American Journal on Addictions. Published by the American Academy of Addiction Psychiatry, 7301 Mission Rd., Suite 252, Prairie Village, KS 66208. Telephone: 913-262-6161. Web site: www.aaap.org.

Many universities operate centers entirely or partly devoted to research in various aspects of alcoholism/addiction. You can find and obtain information from these as follows.

The Rutgers University Center of Alcohol Studies is the pioneer university research center in alcoholism/addiction. It led the effort to have the American Medical Association recognize alcoholism as a disease that could be treated, a policy the AMA adopted in the 1950s. The center today continues research, training, and publication of a leading journal in the field. Its Web site is: www.rci.rutgers.edu/~cas2.

The University of Washington Alcohol and Drug Abuse Institute Library is an on-line library that lists more than seventy-five other centers conducting studies in alcoholism/addiction. Most of them are at American universities, but some are in other countries too. The library's Web site—www.depts.washington.edu/adai/links/catindex.htm—provides links to the home pages of each of these centers.

Three divisions of the U.S. Department of Health and Human Services provide extensive information about current research developments in alcoholism/addiction, much of it on their Web sites:

National Institute on Alcohol Abuse and Alcoholism (NIAAA): http://niaaa.nih.gov

National Institute on Drug Abuse (NIDA): http://nida.nih. gov

Substance Abuse and Mental Health Services Administration (SAMHSA): www.samhsa.gov

Index